Reading Our

T0022269

The Rise of Big
Data Psychiatry

COLUMBIA GLOBAL REPORTS
NEW YORK

Reading Our Minds
The Rise of Big
Data Psychiatry

Daniel Barron

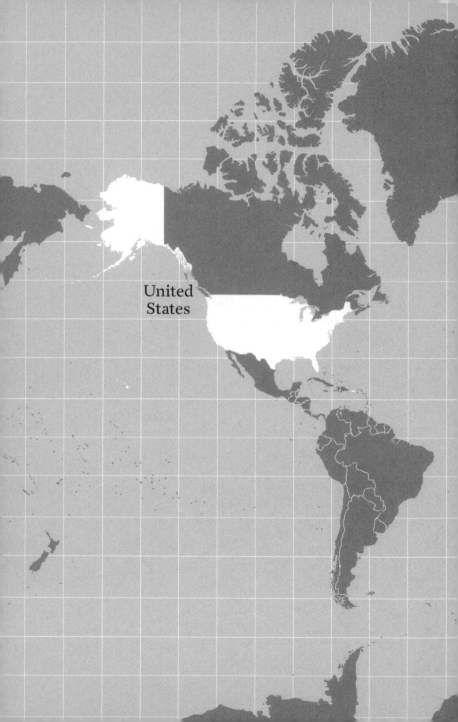

United
States

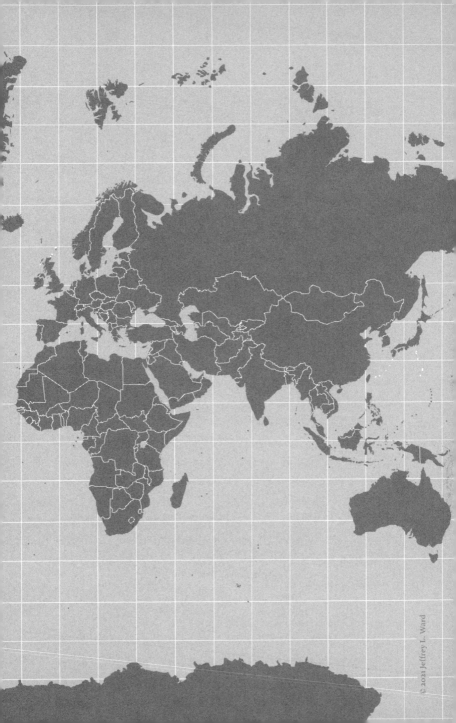

© 2021 Jeffrey L. Ward

Support for this book was provided in part by the Robert Wood Johnson Foundation. The views expressed here do not necessarily reflect the views of the Foundation.

Published by Columbia Global Reports
91 Claremont Avenue, Suite 515
New York, NY 10027
globalreports.columbia.edu
facebook.com/columbiaglobalreports
@columbiaGR

Library of Congress Cataloging-in-Publication Data
Names: Barron, Daniel (Psychiatrist), author.
Title: Reading Our Minds: The Rise of Big Data Psychiatry / Daniel Barron.
Description: New York : Columbia Global Reports, [2021] | Includes
    bibliographical references.
Identifiers: LCCN 2020058016 (print) | LCCN 2020058017 (ebook)
ISBN 9781734420784 (paperback) | ISBN 9781734420791 (ebook)
Subjects: LCSH: Psychiatry. | Mental illness--Diagnosis.
Classification: LCC RC435 .B37 2021 (print) | LCC RC435 (ebook) | DDC
    616.89/075--dc23
LC record available at https://lccn.loc.gov/2020058016
LC ebook record available at https://lccn.loc.gov/2020058017

Book design by Strick&Williams
Map design by Jeffrey L. Ward
Author photograph by Daniel Berman

Printed in the United States of America

For Irene and her mother

CONTENTS

Introduction

It's one o'clock and a seventeen-year-old girl named Irene is sitting beside me in an exam room. Irene is wearing a teal crew neck sweater and cerise corduroys; her brunette hair calmly rests just below her shoulders. She sits with impeccable posture—back straight, hands on her thighs, face calm and expressionless, staring at the wall in front of us. Irene's mother brought her to the hospital because she was having "a psychosis episode."

Since we just met, it's not yet clear whether Irene is psychotic. But as the admitting physician, it's my job to find out. To do this, we'll discuss her clinical history and perform a mental status exam.

The mental status exam is a bedrock tool of a psychiatric assessment. It includes my observations of Irene's body language, speech, and expression in combination with her answers to specific questions about symptoms: what I see and hear paired with Irene's self-report.

Irene and I walk into an adjoining room to speak privately.

"So, can you help me understand what's going on?" I ask.

"Over the last few months, it's been harder and harder for me to concentrate," she begins. Her face remains expressionless; her eyes don't meet mine. I wonder if she is ignoring me or perhaps hallucinating, but she replies to my questions politely and quickly. Perhaps she is depressed or simply shy. She doesn't seem autistic.

She sleeps more and has lost interest in doing essentially everything. Instead she lies in bed all day. She broke up with her boyfriend—whom she tells me she previously loved—because, "well, I was no longer interested."

"Do you ever hear or see things that may not be there? Hear voices or see shadows?" I ask. I remind myself to find a better way to ask if someone is hallucinating.

"Oh, no," she says politely with a reserved shake of her head.

I move on to my standard series of screening questions for schizophrenia, depression, mania, OCD, trauma, and suicide—bits I've memorized from the DSM-5's diagnostic criteria. As we speak, I keep a mental tally of whether what she's telling me fits into one of these diagnostic bins. It doesn't. She doesn't use drugs, has no family history of mental illness, has always done well in school.

I shine a light in Irene's eyes to make sure her pupils constrict—first the left side, then the right. I ask Irene to follow my finger with her eyes as I trace an "H" in front of her head and check that the muscles in her face can smile, frown, bare her teeth, squint, and so on. I test the strength, sensation, and reflexes in her arms and legs. I listen to her heart, lungs, and belly. Nothing seems amiss. Her blood pressure, heart rate, and electrocardiogram are equally normal. Throughout our conversation, Irene is more than calm and cooperative; she is graceful.

12   We return to speak with Irene's mother who tells me that, for the last year or two, Irene has been having "psychosis episodes." Each episode, her mother describes with consternation, lasts two to three weeks; the episodes begin and end without rhyme or reason. During these times, she doesn't sleep but rather just lies in bed, has a warped sense of time, barely eats, and has full conversations with herself that can last an hour. The mother suggests that Irene laughs inappropriately, when no one's around or nothing seems funny.

"I do not, Mom!" Irene protests, breaking character by leaning forward over her legs with an unrestrained giggle. We fall silent: Her giggle is out of place during a psychiatric hospital admission.

Her mother describes Irene's shifting online obsessions: Spotify (Irene felt Spotify was creating playlists to send her messages), astrology (Irene's IP address was blocked from an astrology website for clicking too many pages per hour), and Urban Dictionary (she spends all day reading street slang looking for secret messages in the definitions).

Throughout our conversations, I'm carefully observing Irene: how she sits, whether she moves or taps her foot, where she looks. I consider the types of words she uses and whether her ideas flow one to another. I notice how her facial expression and voice parallel our conversational topic—is she sad when we speak about something sad? These all factor into my mental status exam.

I return to my workroom and, with the help of my electronic medical record's template, enter my mental status exam for Irene:

Appearance: Neat/Clean

Behavior/Attitude: Cooperative, calm

Motor Activity: Hypoactive except, taps her right foot

Gait/Station: Normal

Speech: Normal rate, rhythm, volume, and tone

Mood: "OK" (this is how Irene described her mood)

Affect: Blunted affect. Laughing and lightheartedness,
    which were inappropriate for the context of our
    conversation.

Relatedness: Poor

Thought Process: Normal

Delusions: None

Suicidal Ideation: Denies

Suicidal Intentions: Denies

Suicidal Plan: Denies

Homicidal Ideation: Denies

Homicidal Intentions: Denies

Homicidal Plans: Denies

Perceptual Disturbances: Denies auditory and visual
    hallucinations

If my mental status exam seems subjective to you, I agree. But this is a standard mental status exam, so standard that to document it, I clicked a series of seventeen boxes within Irene's digital note, most simply a normal-or-no reply.

My report doesn't consist of numbers, but rather labels— speech is "normal" or "rapid," not two hundred or a thousand words per minute. Because these labels are subjective, what strikes me as "rapid" speech might change if I see a patient

14   before or after lunch. Whether I think body language is appropriate (or not) might be at the mercy of my mood or suffer from my implicit bias. And there's the problem of describing—not just in prose, but in click-boxes—what I observe.

Outside of note writing, much of a psychiatric evaluation takes place in the examiner's brain—in my brain. Diagnosing isn't so much a tallying up of symptoms (e.g., four of five required symptoms gives you a diagnosis of Major Depressive Disorder, something we'll discuss later in this book), but rather forming an idea for what's going on in a patient's life.

The overall structure of the psychiatric evaluation is essentially unchanged from the early 1900s, when Adolf Meyer developed and promoted a systematic way of gathering information from psychiatric patients.* Meyer, the founding director of the Henry Phipps Psychiatric Clinic at Johns Hopkins University, felt that a clinician needed to see beyond diagnosis to understand how an illness emerged in an individual patient and whether and which aspects of a patient's development, relationships, and physiology—something he called "psychobiology"— were related to that illness.

As I interview Irene, I'm trying to get a feel for the texture of her life, for what it's like to *be Irene*. I ask about specific symptoms because I know what to do with this information—I have a rough idea of how I might treat someone with depression, or psychosis, or obsessive-compulsive disorder.

---

* Meyer's method was based on "informed commonsense," wherein a skilled clinician would speak to a patient and, during this conversation, learn what was necessary to create a bottom-up formulation, wherein the clinican could logically see the pieces of a patient's psychology or social environment that meshed with their biology to produce an illness.

Though the term "psychobiology" has gone out of style, the overall idea remains: A thorough exam is essential because any part might prove crucial to helping the patient. Throughout medical school and residency training, I was told that an important part of being a psychiatrist was *listening* to the patient's words, reflecting on how they made me feel, and then pinning down in prose what I observed in my clinical note, which serves to organize and document what I heard and saw. A psychiatrist, I was taught, functioned much like an anthropologist.

"The most essential skills of the physician," George Engel wrote in his 1977 seminal *Science* article on the biopsychosocial model, "involve the ability to elicit accurately and then analyze correctly the patient's verbal account of his illness experience." Applying Meyer's "psychobiology" to all of medicine, Engel reasoned that all physicians (i.e., not just psychiatrists) should understand the patient's narrative, the context within which their disease operates, and their environment. To fully treat someone, I need to sit with them, hear their story, enter their world by following their words and gestures. It made sense until I went to China.

The China Experiment

As a fourth-year medical student, I had the opportunity to travel to Changsha, a city of 7.4 million people in China's vast Hunan province. I was to visit the psychiatry service of Changsha's highly regarded Second Xiangya Hospital, something like the Johns Hopkins of China. I was thrilled to see how mental healthcare functioned in another culture and was paired with Dr. Hao Wei, who at the time was director of the WHO's Collaborating Center for Drug Abuse and Health. My goal was to

16   attend Dr. Wei's clinic and observe how he interacted with patients. There was just one problem: I speak no Chinese.

For three hours, I sat quietly in the corner and kept tallies as Dr. Wei saw well over forty patients (yes, forty is an incredible number for three hours). Because I had no idea what they were saying, I busied myself observing each patient carefully, drafting character sketches in a little notebook I carried. I jotted down how each patient entered the room, the path they took to a little orange chair in the center of the room. I noted the expression on their face, whether they made eye contact with Dr. Wei or stared quizzically (or suspiciously or angrily) at me. I scribbled down what they were wearing and whether their clothes were clean and pressed or dirty and disheveled.

Did the patient stand, sit, slouch during the interview? Was their voice raspy, soft, high-pitched? Did they share speaking time with Dr. Wei or require interruption? Were they still or did they fidget with their hands, clothes, smartphone? And how did Dr. Wei respond to each patient? Did he seem relaxed, frustrated, worried? At the end of the encounter, did the patient understand it was time to leave or did someone have to escort them out?

After each patient, Dr. Wei would lean toward me and ask me what my diagnosis was. Although I had no access to anything he or the patient said, I was shocked that, more often than not, I was right.

From the corner of the room, without understanding a single word of the clinical conversation, my brain had detected a wealth of clinically relevant information. This information was not narrative-dependent, it was not culture- or content-dependent; I spoke (and speak) zero Chinese. Yet I intuitively understood how each patient's behavior related to their diagnosis, even as a fourth-year medical student.*

But intuitions—so often incomplete or simply wrong—make me uneasy. Even though I felt like I could "read" someone's behavior, I wanted to measure what I had observed and to ground my intuitions in data. I wanted data to understand if there were parts of the exam that were too subtle for me to detect, or perhaps things that I'd never thought of looking at. I also wanted to know when and where and why I was wrong.

As I went through my four years of psychiatry residency, I decided to learn as much as I could about measurement, about how I could measure and gather useful data about my patients to better understand and treat them. The following chapters outline what I have learned.

The Science of Medical Science

In the last hundred years, practically every field of medicine has progressed in immense and unforeseeable ways, largely by the development of clinical technologies. As if by magic, neurologists can now peer into the center of a person's brain to detect a stroke or aneurysm or tumor. Neurosurgeons map where essential brain functions like speech and finger coordination and sight reside, allowing them to avoid and thereby preserve these areas during an operation. When my father-in-law had a brain aneurysm, in a matter of minutes a neurosurgeon snaked a wire

---

* Most people have this skill set: As you walk down the street or sit on the subway, you can probably intuit whether one of your passersby is depressed, or psychotic, or intoxicated. If your partner calls you, even without seeing their face, you can probably tell in the first few seconds what kind of mood they're in. Same concept.

18   from an artery in his groin all the way to the aneurysm's precise
location in his brain, sealing the problem. Fifty years ago, such
an operation would have been impossible; five hundred years
ago, that surgeon would have been proclaimed a wizard.

Infectious disease is no longer guesswork—viruses are
now recognized by their genetic code, which can (in ideal conditions) be identified in a matter of hours and used to build vac-
cines, which can, in turn, be tested and distributed worldwide
in a matter of months. Meanwhile, bacteria are plucked from a
patient's blood, cultured, and countered with specific antibi-
otics. Cardiology, oncology, nephrology, immunology, essentially all modern medical specialties and subspecialties, have
emerged from what was previously simply "medicine." If a
patient in 1920 arrived at a hospital reporting they had chest
pain, the 1920 patient's workup, treatment, and outcome would
be drastically different from a patient's in 2020.

And yet psychiatry has remained largely immune from this
progress. With the exception of some twenty-first-century
jargon, Irene's workup at a psychiatric hospital would have not
looked different from a workup in 1920. Although psychiatry
has found progressively cleverer ways to lump and split their
diagnostic categories, these categories rely almost without
exception on a single diagnostic tool: the psychiatrist's brain.

Psychiatry doesn't function as a medical science. What this
means can be understood by considering how medical science
has worked in cardiology and oncology.

At the close of World War II, President Franklin Delano Roosevelt died unexpectedly. According to those around him,
Roosevelt's health had been in decline since 1940. A heavy

chain-smoker, Roosevelt had gone to the Bethesda Naval Hospital (near the recently established National Institutes of Health) and was diagnosed with hypertension, congestive heart failure, and likely coronary artery disease—a combination of which would occasionally cause him chest pain.

These diagnoses were primarily based on clinical observation: A skilled clinician had spoken with and evaluated Roosevelt and, based on this interview, diagnosed him. Compared to modern tools and assessments, Roosevelt's doctors had little more than folk wisdom at their disposal. And because Roosevelt didn't appreciate the severity of his condition, he largely ignored the few recommendations he received as his health silently continued to decline. Recall that even the diagnosis of "hypertension" was hazy—methods for measuring blood pressure existed, but it was unclear which blood pressure was considered "healthy" (the standard for "healthy" systolic blood pressure was one's age + 100, meaning that in an eighty-year-old, a blood pressure of 180/120 would have been "healthy," a pressure that today meets criteria for malignant hypertension).

In February 1945, Roosevelt returned from the Yalta Conference with Stalin and Churchill, and his staff noticed that he looked frail and thin—observations that were kept secret from the public. In April, he sat for a portrait and began to have a "terrific" headache. He slumped forward in his chair and, hours later, was declared dead from a massive intracerebral hemorrhage.

Tragedy often catalyzes progress and, vowing to better understand a disease that had taken their wartime hero, Congress set aside a historic amount of money to study and combat cardiovascular disease. A group of physicians and scientists representing the world's foremost experts gathered to plan

20   their attack. To combat cardiovascular disease, they deter-
mined, they would study the entire city of Framingham, Mas-
sachusetts, and carefully measure what happens as previously
healthy people develop cardiovascular disease. There was, however, one problem: No one knew what to measure.

It was clear that cardiovascular disease was complex. But
it was unclear which data might unravel this complexity. Scattered clues were beginning to emerge. Scientists had begun to
develop instruments that could measure lipids and cholesterol
in the blood, leading to heated debates about what these measures meant. An early form of the electrocardiogram (EKG) was
rumored to be able to detect heart disease *before, during,* or even
after a heart attack—a revolutionary notion as heart attacks were
thought to be invariably fatal and diagnosed only on autopsy.
Although many instruments were being developed, they were
still in their infancy. Clinicians held to their tried-and-true
methods of evaluating patients and then reaching a diagnosis
based on their clinical acumen, something that varied widely
across clinicians.

In the absence of a clear way forward, the study organizers
decided to measure everything they could think of as rigorously
as possible. The organizers combined exquisitely detailed oral
histories with equally detailed physical exams, a comprehensive
panel of lab values, and a list of clinical tests that slowly grew.
At the beginning, the study organizers identified eighty measures that, collected over time, quickly added up to hundreds
of measures per person. Across the entire city of Framingham,
the researchers began to build an enormous dataset, the size
of which was previously unheard of in medical science (recall,

this was still the pre-computer era, when calculations were performed by slide rule).

The Framingham Heart Study, as it became known, effectively heralded the Big Data approach in medical science: If you don't know what to do, measure everything as rigorously as possible and let the data guide you. I spoke with Dr. Daniel Levy, who (as of 2020) directs the ongoing Framingham Heart Study and has written extensively about the study's history. When I asked how the original study organizers settled on eighty values, Levy told me candidly, "We were just lucky . . . the low-hanging fruit was right there ready to be picked just by making a few simple measurements. [Those measurements] turned out to be useful for diagnosis, for population screening, for following the natural history of disease, and for providing therapeutic insight. We were lucky." So much of science depends on rigorously calibrating an experimental design to invite serendipity.

Although people often conflate Big Data with complexity, Big Data reduces complexity. Because the Framingham Heart Study organizers did not know exactly where to look to unravel heart disease, they gathered hundreds of measurements per person with the hope that they could prune the hundreds down to a handful of the most clinically useful. And they were "lucky." After nearly two decades of gathering data, the Framingham Heart Study indicated that smoking, blood pressure, and cholesterol were three important risk factors for heart disease.

Without question, looking at only three risk factors misrepresents the complexity of heart disease—but, it turns out that it is a useful simplification, one that suggests specific treatments to mitigate disease risk. In fact, after the Framingham

22   Heart Study identified these three risk factors, the field developed specific treatments to address them: smoking cessa-
tion programs, anti-hypertensives for hypertension, statins
for cholesterol. Today, if you go to your cardiologist, they will
ask you whether you smoke, measure your blood pressure, and
check your cholesterol levels, all with the goal of minimizing
your risk of heart disease: personalized medicine.*

While Big Data can help us simplify a complex problem
like cardiovascular disease, it can also indicate that diseases we
think are simple are not necessarily so. Consider how oncologists once viewed cancer.

For centuries, cancer diagnosis (and therefore treatment) was
based in anatomy. Unchecked tissue growth was called cancer;
unchecked tissue growth in the breast was called breast cancer.
This seemed simple, straightforward, but treating cancer was a
capricious enterprise: Two breast cancer patients given the same

* Another way to view the success of the Framingham Heart Study is
through the lens of objectivity, as described by Lorraine Daston and Peter
Galison in their book *Objectivity*. Before the Framingham Heart Study,
physicians treated patients largely based on their clinical observations and
resultant impressions, all of which attempted to capture what happened
in the patient with as high fidelity as possible, something Daston and
Galison call "truth-to-nature." But the advent of clinical sensors like the
sphygmomanometer, immunoassays, and mass spectrometry allowed clinicians to detect and measure things that were previously invisible. This
stage, which Daston and Galison call "mechanical objectivity," is the hallmark
of progress in medical science. Once mechanical objectivity has entered
a medical specialty and once specific measures are proven to be useful in
diagnosis or treatment, the specialty progresses to "trained judgment,"
wherein a clinician incorporates objective measures like blood pressure,
cholesterol level, or EKG patterns into their clinical assessment. Within this
framework, psychiatry remains in the "truth-to-nature" phase of scientific
development. What I describe in this book are digital tools that can produce
"mechanical objectivity" which, hopefully, will lead to "trained judgment."

treatment might have very different responses; a patient might
initially respond to a treatment only to succumb months later.

In the same way the sphygmomanometer revealed the inner
workings of the cardiovascular system, the advent of tools to
study the types of cells present in a cancer (something known
as histology) indicated that cancers found in different parts of
the body might, in fact, be composed of similar or even identical
types of cells. If a cancer from the breast metastasizes to the
lungs, the origin of the metastasis can be identified by the type
of cells it contains. The more recent development of molec-
ular sensors further showed that "breast cancer" was really a
mixed group of cancers, some of which had similar mutations
in key genes and proteins. Ironically, the cell type and mutations
seen in some breast cancers were also found in ovarian or pros-
tate cancer, turning the specificity of anatomy-based diagnos-
tics on its head. Although cancer found in breast tissue remains
popularly known as "breast cancer," this term is progressively
less useful to an oncologist, who reduces the cancer to a specific type of cell or even a specific genetic mutation like BRCA-2,
which then guides molecular-based treatment.

Another example is the HER-2 mutation. When detected
in a cancer found in breast tissue (i.e., not simply a "breast
cancer"), the HER-2 mutation indicates that this specific cancer
will respond to the chemotherapy Herceptin.

So cardiologists and oncologists developed tools and
designed studies to help them measure and reduce the body's
complexity to something understandable, to something that
guides their clinical work. It's important to note that these
technologies did not fundamentally change the way cardiologists and oncologists interact with patients. Bedside manner,

24   empathy, and a human touch are just as important now as they
        were five hundred or two thousand years ago. Clinicians still
        see patients and make decisions about what, where, and when
        to treat. Technology allows clinicians to see what they cannot
        and to include data into their clinical reasoning that they oth-
        erwise could not. Technology allows clinicians to use a "med-
        ical model" to make precise decisions, to better understand and
        treat a patient's illness, to objectively prove to ourselves that
        we're acting in our patient's interest.* In sum, it allows human
        beings like myself—with all my personal limitations and biases
        and inadequacies—to be better clinicians.

        Psychiatry as a Medical Science
        Psychiatry does not function as a medical science. As I'll
        describe in the following chapters, when I see patients, I have
        no instruments to guide and assist and refute my clinical judg-
        ment. Psychiatry remains far behind other medical specialties
        in its use of technology.

        * The claim that psychiatry adopted a "medical model" with the release of the
        DSM-3 in 1980 requires further thought. DSM-3 and all other taxonomies
        of mental disease rely on the clinician accurately understanding and
        representing what's happened in the patient's life. Although psychiatrists
        agree that mental illness has biologic causes and prescribe biology-altering
        therapies and pharmaceuticals to treat mental disease, this alone does not
        constitute a "medical model." The medical model is a way of approaching
        illness through rigorous measurement. In our historical moment, mechanical
        objectivity (instrument-guided quantification) remains the dominant way
        to record and evaluate facts, which is why in 2020, the medical model and
        medical science apply rigorous measurement to evaluate, diagnose, and
        treat patients. Within Daston and Galison's framework, described in the
        preceding footnote: Although psychiatric research is attempting to create
        "mechanical objectivity" to fortify "trained judgment," clinical psychiatry
        languishes in "truth-to-nature" phase of scientific development.

Because I don't have instruments to precisely measure my
patients' concerns, I am forced to rely on my clinical impressions,
on my intuition. Without these instruments, I treat the brain
much the way cardiologists treated the heart or oncologists
treated cancer over a hundred years ago: I speak with a patient
and, based on this story, try to get an intuition for what's going
on in their body.

Unlike in heart disease, where a cardiologist will repetitively
measure blood pressure to ensure that an anti-hypertensive
is having the desired effect, I have no quantitative measures
to determine whether and how much my treatments work: An
antipsychotic "works" if a patient *looks and feels* less psychotic.*
And because I can't connect the way my patient looks and feels
with specific neurons or receptors, I can't prescribe treatments
to alter those neurons and receptors with any reasonable precision. Perhaps, as was the case in breast cancer, the way I'm
thinking about mental illness is not fully correct or, worse, is
completely incorrect. These are all *testable* questions, ones that
medical science can answer.

In this book, I describe a series of technologies that might
dramatically elevate the practice of psychiatry—by measuring
what's on our mind, where we are, what we're doing, and how
and what we say. Each of the technologies already exists and,

---

* Or, as Dr. Kristin Budde (my wife, who is a Yale-trained inpatient and
emergency room psychiatrist, currently working at the University of
Washington) told me in a Catch-22-esque manner, "This week, when a
patient seemed to look worse, one of my colleagues suggested, 'Maybe him
looking worse is actually him getting better.' That's literally an argument I had
with somebody this week! Psychiatry." The absence of quantitative data left
no way for two fully trained psychiatrists to determine or agree on whether a
patient's worse-looking clinical state was evidence of clinical improvement.

26   right now, is being used by Big Tech companies to understand
      our likes and dislikes with the goal of selling products. And yet,
      psychiatry has remained apart from this data revolution even
      though the technology exists and might make a big difference if
      it were used.

      The goal of this book is not to fundamentally change the
      way psychiatry is practiced—even with technology, empa-
      thetic clinicians will still meet with and care for their patients.
      Instead, I hope that this book will show where and how dig-
      ital technologies can improve patient care by shoring up clin-
      ical judgment with quantitative measures. I further hope to
      encourage clinicians and policymakers and patients to reap-
      propriate technologies that they are probably already using and
      have in their pockets and allow these technologies to bolster
      mental health care. I'm aware that, given understandable con-
      cerns about "surveillance capitalism," my suggestion that psy-
      chiatrists and patients embrace digital measures to trace and
      treat patients might bother some people. But please bear with
      me and I'll address these fears.

      To help readers gain an intuition for how and why each
      technology would benefit my work as a psychiatrist, I'll sculpt
      each chapter around the true clinical case of a young woman I
      evaluated and treated, whom you met earlier as Irene.

Online Behavior
Search History and Social Media

Irene's mother, a careful guardian, observed how Irene began to say and do progressively more unusual things—not unusual for everyone, but unusual for Irene. Irene's mother understood that Irene's behavior had a typical pattern, that there was a rhythm to the way Irene conducted her life. Because Irene's mother was familiar with and attentive to this pattern, she noticed when this pattern began to change.

Clinicians understand this intuitively; it's our job to observe the ebb and flow of a patient's mind. Yet researchers tend to study mental illness as an on-off function. Someone is either sick or not sick, depressed or healthy, psychotic or sane. By design, psychiatry's diagnostic bins do not permit gradations: An insurance company wants to know whether you have schizophrenia or you don't. Unfortunately, this bookkeeping formality has pigeonholed our scientific understanding. Our clinical studies (and the statistical tools used to perform them) consider patients as binary disease groups, instead of as continuous gradations of mental states.

28   Each of us has a pattern to our behavior. We are creatures of
habit. We take the same route to work, shop the same stores, purchase the same things. This is called our behavioral baseline—
which is to say, our routine.

Understanding someone's behavioral baseline becomes
relevant to me, a psychiatrist, because someone typically con-
tacts me only after their baseline changes. Perhaps they took a
new route to work and then stopped going entirely. Perhaps they
began shopping endlessly and buying far too much. It's not at
all unusual that a patient is oblivious to these changes: In their
mind, they've been choosing their routes, stores, and purchases
just as always. In their mind, a deviation from their baseline (a
concept most people have never considered) is justified, they
are at the helm of their mind just like any other day, and their
actions are things they *wanted* to do.* So, it's not unusual when
I ask a patient, "What's gone wrong?" that my question is met
with blank stares: They often aren't aware anything is amiss.

---

* If we consider this idea too long, it dawns on us that if we have a pattern to
our behavior—one that can be measured and traced and even predicted—
then we are not really as complex or as free as we would like to believe.
The *New York Times* article tracing a person's steps over a number of
weeks wasn't so much terrifying as it was banal ("Your Apps Know Where
You Were Last Night, and They're Not Keeping It Secret," by Jennifer
Valentino-DeVries, Natasha Singer, Michael H. Keller, and Aaron Krolik,
December 10, 2018). Surely, there's something awfully depressing about
knowing that you—somewhat like a hamster in a wheel—circle through the
same routes day after day and that your behavior is predictable. One of my
favorite parts from the HBO series *Westworld* is the conversation about how
the first attempt to program an artificially intelligent robot (which looks,
acts, reasons, and emotes like a human being) was overly complex and failed.
"The copies didn't fail because they were too simple, but because they were
too complicated," one of the original programmers explained. "The truth is
that a human is just a brief algorithm—10,247 lines. They are deceptively
simple. Once you know them, their behavior is quite predictable."

There is also the patient who *feels* that something has gone
awry in their mental life, but they can't say what. Someone
might come to the emergency room because they feel "depressed
and can't do it anymore," but they can't tell me precisely when
or why they began feeling this way.

It's difficult for me to trace a complete stranger's baseline. I could barely describe my own. Yet each time I see a new
patient like Irene, my goal is to understand something of that
baseline and describe the events that resulted in my clinical
care—whether in the outpatient setting, where I see patients
with chronic mental health concerns, or in the inpatient setting, where I see patients with acute concerns.

Physicians call this tracing of a patient's behavioral baseline—and the deviation from it that brought the patient to a
clinical setting—the "history of the present illness."

In Irene's case, she was an otherwise healthy young lady who
went to class, did her homework, had a boyfriend, and spent too
much time on the internet. Irene folded her own clothes, kept
her room clean—all the mundane things you might expect, so
mundane that it's easy to overlook how crucial her mundanity
was to her clinical picture. Baseline matters.

Coaxing a patient into describing their baseline—their typical pattern—can be a heavy lift. We are notably poor historians
of our conscious lives. In fact, the field of cognitive behavioral
therapy exists for the explicit purpose of helping people consciously recognize and keep track of their emotional, conscious
state in the present moment—which says little or nothing
about the past.

Even with the words we commonly use to describe what our
emotional state is, we may still not have access to the signal of

30   interest. Consider someone's blood pressure—anyone who's had an argument might have a sense that their blood pressure is rising, but we would never expect a patient to keep a journal of how their blood pressure changes throughout the day by intro-specting and jotting down "high" or "medium-high." Such terms would also not be very useful.

Coaxing a patient into describing their baseline from six months ago is even more difficult. Off the top of your head, can you remember how you were feeling six months ago? What about twenty-two weekends ago? Could you say what you were thinking and whether this was different from, say, eighteen weekends ago?

Whether due to the nature of mental illness or simply because they can't remember, people are often unable to provide this level of detail. It's so rare that psychiatrists regularly seek out what we call "collateral," or supplementary, information from family, friends, or other clinicians that might be helpful in understanding a patient's baseline. But secondhand history taking is often hit-or-miss: helpful when it's helpful, not when it's not. If you can't remember what *you* did or said six months ago, why would you remember this about someone else? Not everyone has a mother like Irene.

Fortunately, there is an entire industry formed around measuring, tracing, and preserving a person's behavior—their online behavior.

The Technology

Tech gurus mark 2014 as a turning point in the history of tech-nology. Since 2014, there have been more active smartphone subscriptions than people on the planet. Young adults like Irene now use smartphones at a rate of 85 percent—a statistic that is only expected to increase.

Our lives are progressively more digital. We shop and explore and emote online, whether alone, with our friends, or in a group of complete strangers. The cumulative data produced during our online posts, emoticons, search history, and conversations with our favorite bot is sometimes called our "digital exhaust," but really, this data is the very ore upon which companies like Google and Facebook have built empires. Tech companies are keen to understand (and profit from) how we think, so they vigilantly record which websites we visit, how long we stay, and what we do there. Digital exhaust is the basis of targeted advertising: Follow the breadcrumb trail of someone's digital mind, learn where the crumbs most often fall (i.e., someone's baseline), and then systematically divert foot traffic toward an online marketplace. Unfortunately, these technologies have not yet had an impact on clinical practice.

Nowcasting, a Numbers Game
Google and social media have proven to be enormously accurate (and lucrative) data sources that show what people—both *en masse* and on the individual level—are thinking in the moment, in the now, something known as nowcasting.

Every second, forty thousand people Google something. That translates to 3.5 billion searches per day and 1.2 trillion searches per year. And each day, 1.2 billion people log onto Facebook and 126 million people log onto Twitter, in both cases to record what they are thinking, doing, feeling. They also respond to what their friends were thinking, doing, and feeling—not simply with words, but with pictures, emoticons, and geo-stamped

32   events. This data is time-stamped, a moment-by-moment digital diary.* This data is also backed up, organized, and maintained online so its memory never fades, succumbs to recall
bias, or is forgotten.

Nowcasting uses a technology known as *natural language
processing*, which is a branch of artificial intelligence that presents human language (i.e., words) in a way that machines can
measure and find trends in it (i.e., with numbers). These trends
can tell us something about what people are thinking about or
even what emotions people have toward a particular subject.

For example, if we want a computer to tell us whether people
on Twitter are thinking about cats, we need to present the
Twitter posts in such a way that a computer can make sense of
and then tell us humans something useful about them *en masse*.
One way to do this is to simply list out and tally up the words
used across tweets, something known as "term frequency."

Asking a computer to tell us how many times "cat" is used
across a million tweets gives us a way to calculate "term frequency." But we can take this one step further and make sure
that a handful of tweeters haven't biased our statistic. If we
know that "cat" was used four hundred times, we need to make
sure that ten cat aficionados haven't just repeated the word "cat"
forty times each tweet. To do this, we find the number of tweets
that mention "cat" at least once, creating a measure called "term

* In addition to the actual words someone uses, the way someone types a
word (quickly, slowly, sloppily) and the way someone navigates a website
(nimbly, clumsily) are also useful indicators of someone's mental state and
are being investigated as surrogate measures of reaction time, memory,
and attention—all of which are relevant to mental health and, of course,
marketing.

frequency times inverse document frequency." This allows us to see how many times each unique word is used across all tweets, which is to say, of the million tweets we looked at, four hundred tweets mentioned "cat" at least once. To see how an idea spreads across the Twitterverse, we could further see which unique terms are used by unique users and how an idea spreads across GPS-tagged users.

Nowcasting draws on all of these measures to calculate things like how *viral* a specific idea is. If the frequency of "cat" suddenly spikes across Twitter users—especially if it's being tweeted about by a higher percentage of unique users than other terms—we say that "cat" has gone viral. This isn't an ephemeral phenomenon, but rather a specific measure that can be traced across time.

In addition to measuring what people are tweeting, another method for understanding what's on people's minds is measuring what people are searching for on Google. Dr. Seth Stephens-Davidowitz, a data scientist who has studied what Google searches reveal about our inner lives, noted that, "Google was invented so that people could learn about the world, not so researchers could learn about people. But it turns out the trails we leave as we seek knowledge on the internet are tremendously revealing."

During the COVID-19 pandemic, Google searches for symptoms like "I can't smell" were almost perfectly correlated with state-level reports of disease prevalence. By pooling one symptom with other common searches, researchers could derive a digital symptom profile and watch how it rises and falls over time and across the country. Essentially, they could nowcast the

34 emergence of COVID outbreaks. Google searches for COVID symptoms proved to be so helpful that public health officials used them to guide their attention to regions with likely outbreaks.

People Google advice not simply for COVID, but also when they need to find a job, plan a vacation, or vote in a presidential election. It turns out that among the top ten questions pregnant women in the United States ask Google are whether they can "eat shrimp," "drink wine," "drink coffee," or "take Tylenol." I was fascinated by the intimacy with which people approach their Google search bar.

I mentioned to my wife the top ten questions pregnant women ask and wondered out loud why they didn't just ask their doctor.

Without pausing, my wife rolled her eyes and announced, "You don't want to be judged! You don't want your doctor to even think you're thinking about drinking!"

It turns out she had Googled the same questions when she was pregnant—even though she is, herself, a physician. Just to be sure.

People have enormous (some might say misplaced) trust in Google. It is almost as if people treat Google like a close friend or trusted relative, an Uncle Google that they can ask their most private questions without fear of reprisal or judgment— someone with whom they can peruse ideas and expect accurate advice.

If the study of pregnant women is any indication, people trust Google more than they do their own doctor. Trust is especially relevant to mental health because if people don't trust me, I can't get the information I need to make a sound clinical decision.

Suicide is an especially problematic example. A common
clinical tool is the Columbia Suicide Severity Rating Scale, a
series of templated questions that clinicians ask their patients
to understand (and measure) the patient's risk of suicide. This
type of clinical intervention presupposes two things: 1) that
the patient will answer every question honestly and 2) that the
patient actually knows what they are thinking and feeling, even
if they are in the midst of an emotional cyclone.

A recent study showed that Google searches for explicitly suicidal terms were better able to predict completed suicides than conventional self-report measures of suicide risk.
Perhaps this is because people who are "really gonna do it" go
through the planning and researching (i.e., on Google) of how to
kill themselves, but it could also be that people are more honest
when they approach Google with what's on their mind.

So people use the internet and leave a breadcrumb trail of
their mood, thoughts, and interactions with other people—all
things that are directly relevant to my practice of psychiatry.

When I evaluate a patient, I want to know how they communicate with other people, what they do in their spare time,
and, in a larger sense, how they navigate and think about the
world—not simply in relation to their family and friends, but
in general. How do I learn this? The same way you understand
what I'm communicating: You look at my words.

Social media is an ideal platform to learn how people
interact with the world. Multiple studies have shown something obvious: What we write on social media is indicative of
our mental state. The difference between what I listen for during
a clinical interview and what an algorithm would look for across
a series of Twitter or Facebook posts is that the algorithm is

36   more accurate, has access to more data, and (unlike me) doesn't get thrown off by being grumpy, tired, or hungry.

As Olga Khazan recently observed in the *Atlantic*, "For some people, posting to social media is as automatic as breathing. At lunchtime, you might pop off about the latest salad offering at your local lettucery. Or, late that night, you might tweet, *'I can't sleep, so I think I'm just going to have a glass of wine'* without a second thought."

This is all rich data that can be used to understand something about someone's mood in the moment or their emotional baseline across time.

In a fascinating study, researchers at the University of Pennsylvania looked across over 400 million tweets from users in Pennsylvania. Of these 400 million, nearly 26,000 users (with 46 million tweets) had a least one post with the word *lonely* or *alone*.

According to their report, published in the *British Medical Journal*, people whose posts included the words *lonely* or *alone* were more likely to mention a difficult relationship, that aching hip, substance use, or even poor diet and sleep habits. By using the natural language processing tools I described above, the researchers also noted that people who felt lonely and alone were also more likely to use words associated with anger, depression, and anxiety.

Then the researchers performed a very clever analysis: They wanted to see if the way people expressed themselves indicated a form of baseline emotional state. To do this, they evaluated whether the overall emotional baseline of people's tweets could be used to predict whether they were more likely to be lonely or alone. They discovered that, indeed, they could predict mentions of loneliness with 86 percent accuracy based on the other language a person tweets.

When I spoke with Dr. Sharath Chandra Guntuku at the University of Pennsylvania, I was surprised by how easily his algorithms could pick up on someone's emotional baseline, simply by looking at their tweets.

"It takes only four hundred to five hundred words to pick up on someone's emotional baseline and to be able to predict that baseline better than chance," he told me. That's ten tweets. Of course, this doesn't have a perfect accuracy (just "better than chance") but consider that, in the clinic, I have literally zero accuracy since I don't have access to this data. In a world where every data point counts, the more data I have, the better.

With an understanding of someone's baseline, Dr. Guntuku looked for trends in how this baseline shifts. Because tweets are time-stamped, he could also learn when people were more likely to post about loneliness. As expected, it was in the evening or at night.

What I like about this study is how obvious the conclusions are. Of course people who feel lonely and alone are more likely to experience anger, depression, and anxiety. And, of course, these feelings are more poignant at night, when the lonely and alone are more likely to be so (because they're away from colleagues and friends). This all aligns with our intuition of human nature, but instead of trusting an informal judgment that can be biased by any number of factors, using tweets provides us an objective way to measure and trace and test what we intuitively understand. It provides me a potential tool in the clinic to measure someone's emotional baseline—something that, right now, remains opaque.

38   Forecasting a Change from Baseline

Clinicians typically see a patient once their baseline has changed; people at their baseline level of health—almost by definition—do not come to the clinic or present for admission to a psychiatric hospital. Consider what Irene's mother told me about Irene's internet usage. In the weeks before I saw Irene, Irene's mother said she had begun sifting through Spotify (an online music site); not listening to music, but rather studying songs for secret messages meant only for her.

Irene also began to comb through a specific astrology site, clicking through hundreds of pages per hour. Irene's mother thought this was odd—something she hadn't seen Irene do before. It was so odd, in fact, that the astrology site took notice. Irene clicked on so many pages per hour (and left them open in different browser tabs) that she crashed the website. Perhaps thinking that Irene was a hacker, the astrology site banned Irene's IP address.

Being banned from the astrology site only shifted Irene's obsession to Urban Dictionary—a crowdsourced dictionary for slang words and phrases, something of a Wikipedia for language. Ever vigilant, Irene's mother continued to poke her head into Irene's room multiple times per day and found Irene glued to her computer, the Urban Dictionary page open, hoping to discover some clandestine clue.

The information about Irene's obsessions was critical for my clinical assessment: If Irene's mother hadn't noticed and told me about this behavior, it would have remained for me a clinical unknown unknown.

Irene was unwell, but not clearly so—she still showered and impeccably dressed herself and cleaned her room. Irene sat at her computer calmly, with obsessive focus. If I had walked by her in a library or coffee shop, I might have seen her at her laptop and continued walking. Or I might not have noticed her at all.

Irene's mother understood that there were baseline patterns for internet use—not simply across the population at large, but specific to Irene—and that Irene had deviated from her own "normal" pattern.

But to be clinically useful, this sort of maternal intuition must be measured and tested and proven. (The history of medicine is replete with intuitive but false theories.) This is a question that's fascinated Dr. Munmun De Choudhury.

Since 2006, Dr. De Choudhury has been fascinated by the digital traces that people and communities leave behind online. She began her work looking at how people talk about major life events on social media. One of her first topics was childbirth.

De Choudhury noticed that, on learning they were pregnant, her friends announced their pregnancy on social media like Twitter and Facebook. She became interested in whether the way women expressed themselves online was predictive of a serious condition called post-partum depression. Fewer than half of women suffering from post-partum depression report their symptoms to a clinician; fewer than this receive treatment. De Choudhury wanted to test whether—using social media data alone—changes in a woman's behavior during the prenatal to postnatal period could function as a surrogate measure for post-partum depression.

So, De Choudhury collected Twitter posts from 376 women three months before and three months after they announced giving birth. Within this data, De Choudhury noticed patterns in the way these women interacted socially, the types of emotions they expressed, and even the types of words they used. These patterns began before the baby was born and were amplified following the birth.

In 2012, De Choudhury reported that—based on the three months of prenatal tweets—she could predict which women would develop significant changes in behavior with 71 percent accuracy. By additionally looking at three weeks of postnatal tweets, this accuracy rose to 83 percent.

In 2014, De Choudhury followed up this work by predicting the diagnosis of post-partum depression (as opposed to simply "significant behavioral changes") by using Facebook posts in 165 women. To validate a diagnosis of post-partum depression, De Choudhury performed six interviews with and administered clinical scales to the women involved in the study. They found that the best predictors of post-partum depression were increased social isolation measured by reduced social activity and posting on Facebook—both of which were changes from a women's prenatal baseline.

De Choudhury has applied this line of research to predict other symptoms of mental illness, including psychosis.

In a study recently published in the journal *Schizophrenia,* De Choudhury and her colleagues wanted to test whether they could understand a person's baseline well enough to predict when they were becoming psychotic.

They looked across nearly 53,000 Facebook posts from fifty-one people who had recently developed psychosis and tried to predict when and whether these people—not as a group, but as individuals—were showing signs of another psychotic episode.

De Choudhury discovered that, just before requiring another hospitalization, these patients began to more frequently post swear words, words that expressed anger, or words that alluded to death. They also began to less frequently discuss work, friends, or health. They even began to refer to themselves differently—more frequently using first-person (I, me, mine) and second-person (you, your, yours) pronouns than before.

Using an ensemble of machine learning classifiers (see Chapter Five for more details on the algorithms), they discovered that by looking at what someone posted on Facebook for just one month, they could predict whether that person would be hospitalized with a specificity of 71 percent.* For a medical test, this specificity is actually quite high—high enough to show clinical promise as a tool that screens patients and prompts clinical follow-up.

I have chosen these studies as exemplars of a growing literature that seeks to demonstrate that the way we interact with our computers reflects our emotional and mental state. Because social media is digitized and time-stamped, we can use it to measure, trace, and quantitatively predict not only someone's

---

* In this scenario, specificity refers to whether the algorithm correctly identified people who *weren't* hospitalized, which it did 71 percent of the time. This also means the algorithm incorrectly identified 29 percent of people as not being hospitalized (what's known as a false negative). Sensitivity refers to whether the algorithm correctly identified people who *were* hospitalized, which was 38 percent—the algorithm wrongly identified 62 percent as being hospitalized. Specificity and sensitivity are useful in cases where an outcome is binary: Someone can either be hospitalized or not. In this case, because the algorithm's specificity is greater than its sensitivity, we could say that it is a "conservative" algorithm, one that errs on the side predicting hospitalization. Whether this is acceptable depends on how you want to use the test. If you want a screening tool to identify people who might need more help, then overpredicting isn't a bad thing—many screening tests in medicine work this way. Incorrectly identifying someone who *doesn't* need help is troubling, but failing to identify someone who *does* need help could be fatal.

42   baseline behavior, but whether they are moving away from that baseline.

Back in the Clinic

Quantitative, highly sampled behavioral data extending back months or years would be immensely useful to me as a clinician. Even though a perfect stranger might walk through my clinic door, I could measure someone's baseline emotional and mental state rather quickly if (with their permission, of course) I had access to their Google history and social media profiles. I could imagine a situation wherein (again, with consent) I could download a patient's entire Google search history and see what they have been interested in for the past few months or years. By looking at someone's Twitter and Facebook feed (not to mention other forms of social media), I could further consider how someone interacts with other people and what they have been thinking and feeling at different times of day—again, for the past few months or years.

How these tools are implemented in the clinic will determine whether they are accepted. When I spoke with Dr. De Choudhury and Dr. Guntuku, it struck me how carefully researchers and clinicians are treading on this fertile clinical landscape. De Choudhury told me: "We obviously want to make sure that we have the best uses of this tool [and that] they're not misused by bad actors. That's where the dialogue with patients is very important, so that we can earn their trust. I think it is important to earn the confidence of patients. Transparency and a candid exchange of what this can and cannot do is very important."

To help patients understand this technology and ask them if they are willing to let their clinician collect and monitor their

data, De Choudhury's group is piloting a "Digital Navigator"
position. A Digital Navigator is someone who would sit down
with the patient and their family, explain what data would be
collected and why, and then ask the patient if they want to be
involved in this clinical intervention. De Choudhury imagines
that the consent form would be on an iPad or laptop and, after
a brief tutorial about digital health, the patient could decide
whether to participate and give the clinician access to their
Facebook or Twitter account.

In this framework, a patient could say how much of their
Facebook data they wanted to share. They could say, "I will only
share the last five years," or, "I will share everything from the
beginning of time since I had a Facebook account." Patients
could also indicate if they wanted to share this going forward.

Guntuku emphasized how, for clinical nowcasting to work,
there must be a therapeutic alliance. People trust Uncle Google—
the faceless algorithm in the cloud—who all along is attempting
to make the patient's life more convenient while turning a profit
by selling a patient's data to advertisers. The key element in psychiatric care is for the patient and clinician to have aligned interests so both can trust and engage digital monitoring. The key,
Guntuku told me, was that "the patient has to have complete
agency here—it's not like someone's trying to be a Big Brother.
So we try to make it simple: what they're sharing, why they're
sharing, and what the outputs will look like in the data."

Based on a careful conversation with each patient, the Digital Navigator would retrieve the agreed-upon data, which would
automatically populate into a dashboard that is then accessible
to whomever the patient gives permission. In the same way that
I look at how a patient's blood pressure or cholesterol level has

44   changed over time, the digital dashboard would summarize a patient's recent behavior and define and measure a patient's baseline over time.

This sort of data has the potential to reframe the clinical interaction by modifying the clinical agenda. I can imagine a scenario where I'm seeing one of my patients who has been diagnosed with schizophrenia. If their social media data indicates that they have begun to use words that talk about death or anger or perhaps have begun to refer to friends or family less, we could discuss why and consider changing some part of their treatment. Having data to refer to would be magnitudes more helpful than simply asking a patient, "So, how's it been going?"

Passive Data

Accelerometer, Geolocation, Call Logs

Irene was never a particularly social girl. She had a small circle of friends and, for just over a year, dated a classmate. When I asked her how close they were, she found it hard to say. "I don't know, we were friends," Irene told me with a shrug.

"They'd come over sometimes, after school or on the weekend," Irene's mother offered.

"How active is Irene?" I asked, changing my approach. I'm still trying to understand what Irene was like six months ago, what her behavioral baseline was before this all began.

Baseline is a fundamental concept in medicine. Especially in psychiatry, there is no fixed line between health and disease, between normal and pathology. We intuitively understand that people are different, that there are extroverts and introverts, that some like comedy and some like horror, that some prefer men, some prefer women. A behavior that might strike Irene's mother as a concerning symptom of disease might, in another person, be a shining character trait.

46   If Irene had been a gregarious extrovert, head cheerleader, or perhaps president of her class, then learning that she hadn't left her room in days would be a concerning change from her baseline, that she had withdrawn from an otherwise flourishing and vibrant social life. But if Irene had always been a loner, aloof and bookish, then keeping to herself might seem as normal as grass on a lawn. To say whether Irene had *withdrawn* and whether this withdrawal was indeed a *symptom of disease*, I need to understand what she had withdrawn from, I need context to articulate why Irene's mother was concerned enough to bring her daughter across the state, to my office. What I'm looking for is a change from baseline that might reflect pathology.

In their classic textbook, *Pathologic Basis of Disease,* Robbins and Cotran define pathology as "the study of structural, biochemical, and functional changes in cells, tissues, and organs that underlie disease . . . pathology attempts to explain the whys and wherefores of the signs and symptoms manifested by patients while providing a rational basis for clinical care and therapy." This definition is largely unchanged since the 1800s when Rudolf Virchow, the father of pathology, encouraged his students to "think microscopically." There is little controversy regarding some pathology: You can diagnose cirrhosis, a liver disease, directly with a microscope and indirectly with proteins found in the blood.

Pathology of the brain and brain function is less decisive. Why? Because normal, microscopically healthy brain tissue can produce an infinitely large number of functions. If the liver is a filter, the brain is a Turing machine: It is a piece of hardware with massive functional capability. It is the hardware that runs the software of consciousness. As in all organs, there is a general, average structure for brain tissue, but there are also healthy variants of normal structure; these allow for the healthy, normal variants in brain function that fuel the engine of evolution and allow the diversity that defines humanity's greatest minds and achievements.

And so my job is complex. I need to detect pathology while permitting variability and, to do this, I need data. Psychiatrists have historically performed poorly at this enterprise.*

Psychiatry is an exercise in diversity, in parsing healthy variability from disease. To fully embrace variability, I need tools to measure and quantify and account for that variability, to trace whether what I'm observing is part of a healthy baseline or is indeed a symptom of disease.

Neither Irene nor her mother could give me a definitive answer for how social or active Irene was. But they agreed that

---

* Without quantitative data to guide decisions, psychiatry has fallen victim to social prejudice and has confounded disease with healthy variability. Consider homosexuality. In 1952, the first *Diagnostic and Statistical Manual* (DSM) considered homosexuality and transvestism types of "Sexual Deviation," listed with pedophilia and sexual sadism. In 1968's DSM-2, homosexuality is still a "sexual deviation," but listed under the subcategory "sexual orientation disturbance." In the DSM-3 (1980), this classification was changed to "ego-dystonic Homosexuality," curiously listed with the differential diagnosis of "homosexuality that is ego-syntonic." Homosexuality was dropped entirely from subsequent revisions, such as the revised DSM-3 in 1980. In 1994, the *New England Journal of Medicine* published a report that summarized the absence of any quantitative difference between homosexuality and heterosexuality in any metric. The rise of quantitative data successfully suppressed the operationalization of prejudice and a desire to weaponize medicine as a form of social control. Data allowed variability to thrive—unfortunately, only after decades of failed attempts to straighten the "sexually deviant" with chemical castration, tubal ligation, hysterectomy, vasectomy, and conversion therapy.

48   a few months before we met, Irene began to feel more and more tired. Progressively, she found herself either at her computer or in bed rather than with her friends. This was different from her baseline—she had played in her school's band and enjoyed a social life. Although not a social butterfly, she was also not a loner.

"Did something happen between you and your friends, perhaps an argument or disagreement?" I asked, wondering if some falling-out or adolescent drama had driven her to distance herself. Nothing. She broke up with her boyfriend—whom she once *loved*—because, "well, I was no longer interested."

Whenever Irene was home, she would cloister herself in her room, on her bed, under the covers. At night, she would sleuth the internet for messages meant only for her. Her attention turned more and more on an inner life that teemed with intrigue and mystery, so much so that her friendships seemed too blasé to nurture. Because her clandestine activities were keeping her up all night, Irene's circadian rhythms (her typical sleep-wake cycle) reversed to the point that she was sleeping most of the day and staying up all night.

Many of the questions I ask during a clinical encounter concern a patient's relationships—whether they have a partner, a family, children; do they feel part of a crowd or religious group; do they find that other people annoy them, want to harm them, love them. How someone answers these questions helps me understand the effect a mental illness has had on someone's life.

It's not surprising that mental illness affects our social lives: A severely depressed patient who remains in bed all day cannot engage in meaningful relationships. Someone in the throes of a paranoid psychosis may understandably find it hard to feel safe around or trust people, even their own family. On the other hand, someone in a manic high might never stop socializing.

As the biopsychosocial model suggests, our social activity is a useful indicator of our mental health. But how would you describe your social life? "Good"? "Fulfilling"? "Exhausting"? Or also, if I were to ask how many hours each week you spend with friends and family, could you tell me? Were you more social this week than, say, twenty-three weeks ago?

Right now, psychiatrists lack tools to measure and trace what we agree is essential clinical data. Instead, we rely on memories and impressions that a patient or family member can offer. We are unable to measure and so are unable to fully define baseline.

We don't remember how much time we spend with others or how active we are because our goal is not to remember, but to act. Unlike tallying our expenses or bills, the vast majority of our lives are lived passively, reflexively, breathing without keeping track of how often or how long.

The Technology

Passive data collection is a relatively new form of biomeasure that, instead of requiring people to respond to questions or engage with a software platform, simply uses a digital device to effortlessly record what someone is already doing. The primary instrument for passive data collection is the smartphone.

The smartphone is the hub of modern social life, perhaps just the hub of modern life. We carry our smartphones every-where. (The only place I don't bring mine is the pool.) We interact with colleagues, friends, and family throughout the day with our smartphones, perhaps more than in person. From our

50 pocket or our purse, our smartphone measures our movements with accelerometers, our location with GPS, and our social engagement with the number of calls and texts we send. Each measure captures a facet of someone's lived experience and can be used to understand someone's baseline lived experience, to understand someone's baseline, and, therefore, to detect when there are changes from that routine that might indicate something has gone awry.

Accelerometers

Activity—formally called psychomotor activity—is a core part of any mental status exam. How much someone moves around my exam room reflects their mental state. I use terms such as "hypoactive" or "hyperactive" to describe when a patient sits motionless in a chair or perhaps cannot sit at all, pacing or wringing their hands throughout a conversation. I am meant to project what such behavior might mean for someone who is outside my clinic. If they can't sit still during a doctor's visit, how could they sit still at work? Or home?

Accelerometers have a long history in psychiatry. An accelerometer is simply a device that measures *acceleration* along an axis, which is to say, movement. The modern accelerometer first began as a variant of the self-winding wristwatch. An early accelerometer was developed in 1976 at the National Institute of Mental Health (NIMH) explicitly to measure movement in psychiatric patients. Advances in sensor technology and computer processing have led to motion-analysis systems that can precisely track and record a three-dimensional position of someone well enough to define how much someone is moving, how fluidly, and even the type of movement (my Apple Watch can tell whether I'm walking, jogging, or swimming—and even my swimming stroke—simply based on my accelerometer data).

To understand how accelerometers are clinically useful, consider childhood ADHD. Early studies of childhood ADHD presented a unique problem: The disorder is often situation-specific; behavioral problems due to hyperactivity may not be present at home or in a clinician's (or researcher's) office. ADHD diagnosis and research rely on impressions and ratings from classroom instructors about how much a child moved about a classroom. Here is an example of one such rating:

Fidgets with hands or feet or squirms in seat.

NEVER	OCCASIONALLY	OFTEN	VERY OFTEN
0	1	2	3

This rating scale asks an instructor to capture a child's hyperactivity *throughout the entire day* in a single, subjective number. Although well-trained instructors could carefully note a child's psychomotor activity, such scales are no substitute for firm quantitative data. Subjective ratings were soon replaced by a cleverly designed seat cushion, which measured when and how much a child fidgeted, tilted, or shifted their weight in their classroom chair. The sensor in the cushion was, unfortunately, biased by a child's weight and size. Another shortcoming of the cushion was a bit more obvious: To work, it required hyperactive children to stay seated, a criterion on one of the clinical scales:

52   *Leaves seat in classroom or in other situations in which re-
maining seated is expected.*

NEVER	OCCASIONALLY	OFTEN	VERY OFTEN
0	1	2	3

An early compact accelerometer—even though it was in a fanny pack—greatly improved our ability to continuously measure movement—not simply on a chair, but around the classroom, playground, and home. The fanny pack could also be worn at night, further providing measurements for how much a child slept.

The accelerometer allowed Dr. Linda Porrino and colleagues to quantitatively demonstrate that children with ADHD were more active than age-matched controls both day and night. Though this hyperactivity was greatest during school, it was not apparent during recess. Porrino also showed that a single dose of dextroamphetamine (Adderall) decreased this hyperactivity by 28 percent, bringing this hyperactivity to normal.

Because Porrino had continuous measurements of the children throughout the day, she could break down precisely *when* children with ADHD struggled the most (reading and math time) and also ensure that medication didn't negatively interfere with times when ADHD kids weren't struggling (recess). Measurement also helped researchers determine the smallest amount of medication needed to produce behavioral improvements—something known as a clinically effective dose. It's useful to note that, even for a caring, expert teacher and clinician, knowing how much and when a child moves around and whether and how much that behavior changes with treatment is not *obvious*; having numbers to supplement clinical judgment proved extremely useful.

Accelerometers are also being used to measure sleep—how many hours total, how many in each sleep stage.

Today, accelerometers are cheap and ubiquitous. You can find them in any smartwatch or smartphone—even in some shoes. Clinicians are progressively less justified in making treatment decisions related to activity or sleep without grounding these decisions in quantifiable data.

Geolocation

Closely related to accelerometer data is global positioning system (GPS) data. Accelerometers measure *how much* movement while GPS measures *where* that movement takes place.

I was surprised to learn that GPS doesn't require a device to *send* any data; it's based on *receiving* data. Each of twenty-four satellites—originally put in orbit and still maintained by the U.S. military—has a highly accurate atomic clock. All satellites' clocks are carefully synchronized and transmit the same time signal at every moment. But because it takes different lengths of time for each satellite's signal to reach your chip (since some satellites are farther away than others), your GPS chip might receive a "4:00" signal from satellite 1 and a "3:59 and 55 seconds" from satellite 2. By comparing the signals from four or more satellites, your GPS chip can triangulate (quad-angulate?) your position based on the known position of the GPS satellites.

All you need to take advantage of this signal is a receiver (to listen) and a processor (to quad-angulate your position). GPS

54   chips are now cheap and ubiquitous, small enough to be on key-chains and precise enough to help me find my keys on my couch by the window, under the cushion.

GPS can tell us where in coordinate space we are, relative to the GPS satellites. By enriching a GPS location with geographic data like the addresses and business names on Google Maps, we can deduce what someone's doing, like grocery shopping, having dinner at a restaurant, or having a happy hour drink at a bar. Pairing a geographic location from the internet with GPS coordinates is called *geolocation*.

In the *New York Times* article "Your Apps Knows Where You Were Last Night, and They're Not Keeping It Secret," reporters were able to access geolocation data from Ms. Magrin, a forty-six-year-old math teacher. Within a four-month period, her smartphone had recorded her geolocation 8,600 times, or roughly once every twenty-one minutes. By mapping Ms. Magrin's data, the reporters produced a lovely visual demonstration of behavioral baseline. From the data, it was obvious which route Ms. Magrin took to her classroom, where she liked to grocery-shop, where her ex-boyfriend lived, where she enjoyed hiking.

Of course, the purpose of the article was to alert the public that Ms. Magrin's data was being collected surreptitiously and sold to marketing companies without her knowledge. Her data was being mined by tech companies for profit. Yet within this same article is a beautiful demonstration of how powerful a similar, HIPAA-compliant sampling might be, one that Ms. Magrin approved of and consented to.

You might imagine that, in Irene's case, geolocation data might have shown months of a normal, baseline activity: Irene going to class, meeting her friends at an ice cream parlor, walking through the park with her boyfriend. But as Irene descended into her psychotic episode, her daily geolocation pattern tightened on her home until, weeks in, her movement was represented by a single dot over her bed during the day and over her computer at night. Such variations can only be detected if there is a clear, quantitative understanding of baseline.

One clever application of geolocation data tackled a long-known problem in chemical dependence: maintaining sobriety. People who want to remain sober are counseled to avoid the people, places, and things associated with their former alcohol or drug use.

After completing an alcohol rehabilitation program, researchers gave patients a smartphone app that tracked their geolocation. When the patient neared a location previously tagged as "high-risk," like a bar or liquor store they used to frequent, the patient would get an alert, a digital reminder that perhaps they should steer clear. With the patient's approval, this alert was also sent to the patient's counselor, allowing further clinical follow-up. Although geolocation data is considered passive data collection, this sort of app is an *intervention* that showed promising results: People who used the app were less likely to drink alcohol.

Call Logs

Traditionally, scientists define human social networks by asking relatively small groups of people (fewer than a hundred) what they thought about their peers. For example, Dr. Nicholas Christakis—a palliative medicine doctor turned network science guru—created a computer platform called Trellis to

56   understand the social networks of entire Honduran villages. Christakis and colleagues interviewed each villager one-by-one and asked them who they liked and disliked, who they went to for advice, and who came to them for advice. By asking standardized, detailed questions, Christakis could tally up how many people liked or disliked, relied on, or avoided any one individual. Transforming a series of questions into numbers allowed Christakis to apply decades of advances in network theory and, in a series of innovative studies, to model how information or disease would spread through this social network.

Christakis's work is noteworthy both for its innovative look at information in society and also for the sheer amount of effort it takes to, in person, interview 5,773 Honduran villagers and churn these interviews into useful quantitative data. Obviously, this isn't an option for me clinically—I can't interview every person in a patient's community to create a map of that patient's social network. But because an estimated 90 percent of people in first-world countries have a mobile phone, I have access to one form of their social interaction: call logs.

Call logs are straightforward. A call log details who and when you called (or who called you) and for how long. The same applies for text messages: who, when, how long. Call logs have value because they present a *measure* for someone's social interaction: who, when, and how much someone interacts with other people within a social network.

Instead of painstakingly interviewing each individual in a community and tracing back their interactions, call logs make use of the data an individual generates naturally over time. In 2007, Drs. J. P. Onnela, A. L. Barabasi, and colleagues built a social network from millions of mobile call logs over an eighteen-week period. The telecommunications company (who provided the call logs) de-identified customers' personal information by randomly assigning a combination of numbers and letters to each log (e.g., Timmy's log was identified as A1B2C3), making it impossible to recover actual phone numbers or other information that could pair an individual with their data.

Because the majority of our social lives takes place by smartphone and is digitized and recorded, it can be used to measure someone's *baseline* social communication and how this baseline changes over time. Instead of my asking patients how close they are to their partner, family, or friends, I could instead get a measure of how much they call or text. Since many mental illnesses change social activity—either decreasing it or increasing it depending on the illness—such digital maps of our social networks and how they change with symptoms could prove to be quite useful.

Back in the Clinic
Irene entered my clinic a complete stranger. I had about an hour to sort out what was going on in her life and create an initial plan of how best to help her.* So I would've embraced any data that could have helped me overcome the blank box that was Irene's life. Each of the data points I've described so far— browsing history and social media in Chapter One; accelerometer, geolocation, and call logs in this chapter—can be found on

* If you think that hour seems like an impossibly short amount of time to piece together someone's clinical history, diagnose, and form a treatment plan, you're right. It is. But the clinical reality is that an hour is a rather long amount of time. Many outpatient clinics have thirty-minute appointments. If I were working in a bustling psychiatric emergency room, I might spend less than thirty minutes triaging and treating a patient.

58   your smartphone. Irene might have walked into my clinic with a smartphone—she could even have handed me her unlocked smartphone and given me permission to analyze her data.

In fact, many patients are willing to offer me any and all information that might help me better understand and treat their illness. But having permission to access all of Irene's data doesn't mean I know how to glean useful information from her smartphone data, especially clinically useful information. Data science is complex, and implementing data science is much more so.

I will discuss implementation in Chapter Five; however, for now, it's useful to consider what would've been helpful to me as I interviewed Irene and was trying to understand how to help her.

After meeting with Irene and her mother, I reviewed her chart history—another doctor's clinical note documenting Irene's recent emergency room visit, a series of laboratory values describing her blood chemistry, her hormone levels, and whether she had correct levels of relevant vitamins. I checked to see if there were any drugs or toxins in her urine that could explain her bizarre behavior. I looked at her electrocardiogram. I did all of this to augment my senses, to be able to see and include otherwise invisible information into my clinical thinking.

I didn't, however, apply the same rigor to Irene's social life, an essential part of the biopsychosocial approach. True, part of my clinical exam focused on Irene's social life. But instead of acquiring *measures* of how often she interacted with her friends and family, I asked her these questions in an almost off-hand manner: "How's your relationship with your friends and family?"

How, *precisely*, was her social life different in the week preceding her admission than in the six months before? Were there periods of inactivity punctuated by bursts of mania? Was there a steady decline in activity from what was otherwise Irene's baseline? These are all answerable questions; questions for which Big Tech companies have answers but I do not.

Conversational Data
What We Say and How We Say It

Irene was unwell, but not obviously unwell. Her mother, con-
vinced that Irene was in the throes of a "psychosis episode,"
recounted specific troubling changes: the delusional internet
sleuthing, the solitary laughing, the isolation from her friends.
Something about Irene was a bit "off," and yet, I struggled to
pinpoint what it was.

During my clinical exam, I paid careful attention to Irene's
face and whether it reflected our conversation. Did her expression match the content of our conversation? Did she smile and
laugh at something funny and appear sad at something sad? Did
she gaze off into space or look at me? Were her changes in expression fluid and coordinated, or were her movements jerky, like
she was twitching a smile? I also carefully noted the words Irene
used and whether her words formed sentences that then flowed
into coherent paragraphs. I observed how she walked to my exam
room, whether she wiggled in her chair, tapped her foot.

Somewhere in my brain, I kept a running tally of what might
or might not have been useful. Twenty minutes before, we were

complete strangers. Now we were in a high-stakes poker game: she, acting normal; me, studying her, looking for meaning in her behavior, waiting for an elusive tell.

Minus her single out-of-place giggle that I mentioned in the Introduction, the clarion tell never came. If I really considered what I'd observed, Irene was *more* than normal; she was poised, graceful. If I had passed her in a park or hallway, I wouldn't have noticed her at all. I wondered if I felt Irene was "off" simply because her mother told me so.

After our conversation, I returned to my workroom to write up my notes and, specifically, organize the results of my mental status exam. The mental status exam is a framework meant to help me organize and operationalize the way I think about a patient's behavior, to help me think through how best to help. But like most clinical frameworks, the mental status exam is only as useful as the information it contains.

In Irene's electronic chart, I clicked a series of tick-boxes to document my observations:

Motor Activity: Hypoactive, except taps her right foot
Gait/Station: normal
Speech: Normal rate, rhythm, volume, and tone

Whether I'm looking at my own or another clinician's, I invariably find the mental status exam scientifically unfulfilling.

Consider the word *normal*—as in, Irene's speech was *normal*. What does normal mean, precisely? In what way is someone or something normal? Further, what does a normal conversation sound like? Of course, if Irene sobbed while telling me a joke, that would be *abnormal*. Or if she looked at the wall instead of

62   my eyes while speaking, that, too, would be abnormal. There seem to be multiple ways to have an abnormal conversation, and yet I can't quite put my finger on what a normal conversation is. Clearly, the very nature of a clinical exam—wherein I poke and prod at someone's mind—is not *normal*.

The mental status exam is inherently subjective and vague. What seems like "fast speech" to one clinician may not seem quite so fast to another. A patient who claims they are in a "good" mood on Monday might give the same report on Friday and yet be in very different moods. (Incidentally, "good"—not "really good" or "kind of good," just "good"—is how more than half of my patients describe their mood, which always strikes me as odd since they are in a psychiatric hospital.)

Language is, some linguists argue, necessarily vague. Vagueness permits conversational wiggle room, an ambiguity that for much of our evolutionary history served a useful social purpose. Because words are vague, we can communicate without requiring that everyone is thinking about the exact same thing: Communication requires we be on the "same page," not the same paragraph or sentence or word.

It's hard to imagine Neanderthals (or Romans or Knights Templar) planning the precise minute and second they'd close in on a hunt. It wasn't until very recently in our history that we had the concept of clock at all, not to mention the notion of seconds. Language evolved to serve a very specific and imprecise purpose: communicating the general idea of a topic. Vagueness allows conversation to be efficient.

Yet, in medicine, vagueness can be fatal. I do not prescribe "a pinch" of Ativan, but a thousandth of a gram; I use carefully calibrated laboratory tests to titrate the thyroid medication levothyroxine down to the *millionth* of a gram. No medication is without side effects, so before I begin any medication, I ought to be sure that I'm pairing—as rigorously as possible—a particular condition with a particular medication dose. If I'm treating someone's hypothyroidism, I would invariably follow this procedure; but when I'm treating someone's depression or psychosis, this is not at all what I do.

Quantitative measurement is a routine, defining feature of every medical science except for psychiatry, whose mental status exam exclusively contains words. "How's your mood?" "Good." What is someone's thought process? "Normal." Besides the lack of precision words offer, the problem with subjective labels is that they communicate a low clinical expectation for precision. With an offhanded exploration of something as critical as mood, I am signaling to my patients that their mood isn't really that important, that a brief, superficial assessment is all I care about. I've often wondered whether my patients believe that I—simply by looking at and listening to them for twenty minutes—can divine the inner workings of their brain. Or perhaps even more troubling, I wonder whether clinicians believe that we can adequately assess the inner workings of someone's brain with a single conversation, or if habit has made us blind to our own vague inadequacy.

Physicians routinely augment our senses with instruments like a sphygmomanometer or stethoscope. We've generally agreed that the heart and lungs are difficult to hear with a naked ear, so it's best practice to amplify our limited sense of hearing with a stethoscope. With the aid of a stethoscope, we no longer *listen* to the heart, we *auscultate* the heart.

64   Auscultation is fundamentally different from listening. I placed my stethoscope on Irene's chest to auscultate the characteristic *lub-dub* . . . *lub-dub* cadence of her heart's atrioventricular and semilunar valves snapping shut. I listened for murmurs, which might portend trouble.

I further ordered an electrocardiogram (EKG) to break down Irene's heart sounds into the specific electrical overtures that spread through her atria and ventricles. I studied Irene's EKG as if reading sheet music, ensuring that the timing, crescendo, and finale of each heartbeat fell in place. I ensured that across her heart, each muscle bundle was in tune and on time down to the thousandth of a second.

But at no point in my psychiatric exam did I auscultate Irene's speech or posture or facial expression. The *lub-dub* of her mind seemed off, but I couldn't quite describe how or why or where. In the same way I'd use an EKG to detect the specifics of someone's heart function, I needed a tool to quantify and trace which words Irene used and when, how her facial expression changed and when, where her eyes glanced and when. In this chapter, I describe a series of tools that could help me auscultate Irene's behavior.

The Technology

Attempts to understand people's spoken and body language extend as far back as society itself. In literature, character development depends on the reader believing and keeping pace with a character's defining words and gestures. We intuitively know that what a person says and does—and how they say and do it—is not only useful data, but essential data, the essence of that person.

In the early 1900s, psychologists presented the first systematic attempts to understand how someone's words reflect their mental state. By 1931, there were 148 scientific manuscripts attempting to understand language in children. Speech was considered a behavioral response to the environment. One author declared, "Speech reactions are primarily to be considered causally or functionally as a response to the total stimulus situation before the reagent." The important child psychologist Jean Piaget thought that speech reflected an individual's social development and served a specific *psychological* function (rooted, of course, in Piaget's theoretical model of the psyche). Speech was understood in the context of its psychological purpose rather than as an entity in itself.

These efforts were not so much aimed at measuring *speech*, but rather, at validating a dominant theory of cognition. They were, in essence, circular: A particular measure was useful if it sufficiently captured some facet of a dominant cognitive theory, which, in turn, indicated what to measure. (As I reviewed this literature, I couldn't help but think about cosmologists fastidiously measuring Earth's distance to the other planets in order to prove that the earth was the center of the cosmos.)

Early attempts to understand the psychological properties of speech (or text generally) floundered not simply because of theoretical blinders, but because of the enormous complexity of the task itself. Without efficient computational power, people tried to make sense of speech with their brains and, unfortunately, ended up telling us more about a dominant theory than the speech itself. Why measurements proved important can perhaps be best understood by first considering the way people walk.

66   Imagine we are people-watching in Central Park at dusk (one of my favorite pastimes). Because the sun is low, we can only make people out by their silhouette. From a park bench, we sit and make up stories about what's going through a person's mind, about what mood they're in, their age, their gender. If we see a silhouette standing up straight and advancing at a clipping pace, we might describe that person as young, happy, and excited. Someone who is slouching and slowly shuffling along might be sad or tired or aged. Silhouettes swaying at the hips might be feminine whereas blockish silhouettes might be masculine. These are our stories, our ideas for how we think people *ought* to walk if they are happy, excited, or masculine. Terms like "blockish" and "sway" are not measurements for how an individual is *actually* walking, but rather words we use to express gendered concepts of brutishness or finesse. (They are mental models for how we perceive the world—more on this in Chapter Four.)

Walking can be measured—not just qualitatively, by our brains sitting at a park bench at dusk, but quantitatively, by a computer. For the last four years, I've been working with the Computational Psychiatry group at IBM to develop tools to measure what we observe from that park bench.

Steve Heisig is a computer scientist, formerly at IBM, who helped me think through ways to explain what our computer algorithms do. These algorithms take a video of a person and automatically label where the head, shoulders, knees, and toes are. With the body parts labeled, the algorithm creates a skeleton image, a stick figure of that person. Now that the silhouette has been reduced to a stick figure, we can measure the movement of the hips relative to the chest and shoulders and head,

how quickly the legs move, and even how much the legs bend
at the knees and arms bend at the elbows at each moment (or
frame) in a step. Each of these measurements provides a vector
(or set of numbers) that captures the body's position at each
moment in space. By comparing vectors across time, you can
measure how someone moves through space.

The face can also be measured. Algorithms can tag eyes,
ears, mouth, and nose, and the distances of each tag relative
to the others can be measured as someone speaks or smiles or
frowns. The face, too, is then vectorized to quantify the position
of each part of the face across time and space.

When the corners of someone's mouth move closer to the
eyes while the middle of the mouth remains relatively static, we
understand this as a smile. How long these distances remain in
this position determines how long someone is smiling. Instead
of saying that a person is "smiling" or even is "happy" (both of
which are based on the assumption that all "smiles" are the same
and, worse, that someone who smiles is therefore "happy"), we
can simply measure how many seconds (or frames) a person's
face held a specific position.

Computer vision software recognizes and labels an object
(eyes, shoulders, knees) and assigns numbers to how those
objects change relative to one another across time. The bril-
liance of this overture isn't to get a computer to tell whether
someone is walking (which is something my toddler could do),
but to vectorize—automatically, without any human input—
the movement itself. Once we have vectorized a phenomenon,
once we have pinned reality down in numbers, we can apply the
full scope of mathematical and statistical tools that have been
developed over the past five hundred years. (Or as Steve told

68   me, "So once you get your data into a vector, there're a gazillion tools that you can instantly use.")

It should be clearer now how vectorizing a phenomenon is immensely powerful: It opens the door to a near limitless type of tasks we can perform with the aid of computers.

Vectorizing speech comprises two general forms: the words and the sounds. This intuitively makes sense—it isn't just what someone's saying, but *how* they're saying it that imbues meaning to our verbal communication. Imagine your friend John calls you on the phone (you can't see John's face so have no access to his body language). You've been friends for a long time, and you have an intuition for how John *normally* speaks—you recognize John's voice by the types of words he typically uses (content) and also by the way he sounds (acoustics). If you ask John how he's doing and he replies with a long, drawn-out sigh, "Ohhh. [*sigh*] I'm . . . well . . . okay," you instantly know that, contrary to what he said, John isn't okay. A combination of what John says and how he says it tells you something is amiss, meaning that something has deviated from John's normal pattern, his baseline.

Whenever scientists try to understand a phenomenon, we begin by surveying a large body of material to create a *normative distribution*. This requires an immense amount of data and, for many decades, analyses of speech were complicated by a lack of a large enough dataset to develop a sufficiently large and generalizable normative distribution. First attempts relied on relatively scant samples collected by an individual research group that were painstakingly transcribed, labeled, and evaluated by hand (or rather, by ear, eye, and hand).

Computers revolutionized linguistic analyses. With the emergence of the internet, we could give computers access to

human language *en masse* through large stores of books, newspa-
pers, or other texts, all of which were readily available online. For
example, since 1971, Project Gutenberg has digitized over sixty
thousand books, which are freely available online. This enormous
training set combined with algorithms that automatically analyzed language provided a blossoming normative distribution.*

In Chapter One, we briefly covered how measuring the frequency of individual words on someone's social media account
allows us to create useful measures of what that person is
thinking about—so much so that such measures can predict
psychosis and suicide. The first step in understanding speech
is to bring *what* someone says into a useful format by creating a
transcript. Natural Language Toolkit is a popular tool that takes
unpunctuated, transcribed speech, and annotates it with additional information based on word choice and order. One of these
annotations is known as parsing.

A speech parser takes "John kicks the ball," and identifies
"John" as the subject noun, "ball" as the object noun, "kicks" as
the verb, and "the" as an article. The parser then groups words
into phrases based on how closely they relate to one another. For
example, "the" and "ball" would be grouped into an object noun
phrase: "the ball."

By parsing language this way, the phrase "John kicks the
ball" is tagged with additional layers of information that tell you
how, based on enormous samples of text (a normative distribution), English-speakers on average group ideas. This additional

---

* It can't be understated how automation progressed the field of language
processing. Jong and Wempe describe how, in a single day, a computer
program they wrote performed a task that would take one person working
full-time eight months.

70   information further allows you to test whether an individual speaker uses longer noun phrases or expresses ideas in a more complex way than other speakers.

By looking across hundreds of millions of words, we can further assign each word a vector based on how often (or how *close*) it is used in combination with other words. Whereas *meaning* is a somewhat nebulous term, *distance* is something we can measure and, importantly, vectorize. If you find it difficult

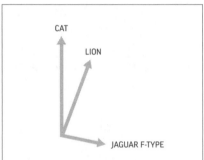

Figure 1. Illustration of how cat, lion, and the Jaguar F-type sports car are related in vector-space.

to understand precisely how this works, you're not alone. A helpful way to build an intuition for how words are vectorized is to think of words' vectors as arrows proceeding from a common point (see Figure 1). Consider the words *cat, lion,* and *Jaguar F-type* (sports car). You might imagine that, of these three words, the cat and lion would be the most similar and so would be represented by vectors that are closer together within our three-dimensional space. The Jaguar isn't entirely different, but is clearly not an animal, so the vector representing Jaguar would be pointing in a different direction. These three words, however, are closer in our three-dimensional space than *ice cream sandwich,* which is something else entirely. Ice cream sandwich would be pointing in quite a different direction from cat, lion, or Jaguar.

By vectorizing individual words, we can automatically build categories based on how close words are to one another within this three-dimensional vector space. For example, lion and cat might fall under the category "feline" or "mammal" whereas Jaguar might be closer to Maserati within the category "sports car." This is another way we can understand the content of someone's speech. Which emotions someone expresses can likewise be measured by determining whether they frequently use words associated with positive and negative emotions. This is similar to the psychological analyses originally thought of in the early 1900s. However, conclusions drawn from such analyses are quantitative and based on massively more data.

Coherence is a way to measure how well one idea flows into another. One way to understand coherence is to construct a speech graph. A speech graph combines the vectors of individual words by essentially stringing them out together. By tracing the path of each word's vectors, you can create a path of someone's speech throughout three-dimensional space and measure how much someone is "skipping around." Speech graphs help identify how organized someone's speech is, which might have helped me detect whether Irene had been disorganized, albeit so mildly I wasn't consciously aware because my brain had filled in the gaps.

In addition to the content of someone's speech, we can further evaluate speech's acoustic properties. The acoustic component of speech comprises the sounds a person makes while speaking. These include the intonations of someone's voice—how monotonous or singsong their voice is (pitch), how long someone pauses between words or syllables to breathe or think,

72   and how many syllables someone says per second. These are things our brains intuitively pick up on—in the same way we were able to tell that John wasn't really okay over the phone, we're also able to tell over the telephone whether someone is out of breath, excited, or even drunk based on the *acoustic* properties of their voice alone. But by vectorizing the qualities of someone's voice, we can perform sophisticated analyses and thereby gain a deeper understanding of it.*

Each of the tools I've described above represents an extraordinary feat of computer science combined with decades of work in mathematics, linguistics, kinematics, and physics—an intellectual tour de force that leverages our progress over the last five hundred years. Just think about it: In my research, I'm able to take a video and measure how fluidly someone walks, the specific way their face moves when they smile and speak, even how and what they're saying. It's so cool it makes me giddy. Now let's see how it could help me in the clinic.

Back in the Clinic

Even though I paid careful attention to Irene's words and body language, I had no way to measure precisely what I saw. Simply *measuring*—even without knowing what those measurements mean in terms of diagnosis or prognosis—could have enormous clinical value.

Right now, I might describe a manic patient's speech in my clinical note as "rapid, loud." With the tools listed above, I could

---

* To get an intuition for how an acoustic analysis works, I encourage you to check out swphonetics.com for an interactive demonstration. See, for instance, https://swphonetics.com/praat/tutorials/understanding-waveforms /speech-waveforms/.

describe a patient's speech as 200 words per minute, a volume of 70 decibels, and a pitch of 180Hz. A further acoustic analysis might tell me that the patient's speech had a median of seven syllables per second. What's cool about this is that I could then compare this number daily throughout this patient's admission to see how it normalizes with treatment. For example, when my manic patient's speech slows to three syllables per second, I know that his speech is more "normal."

It would be difficult to overstate how useful measurements— simple numbers—would be in a clinical setting. These measures are being heavily researched by multiple groups around the world. For example, in 2015, a group of scientists led by Dr. Cheryl Corcoran, then at Columbia University, reported that subtle speech patterns (far too subtle for a clinician to detect) are evident in schizophrenia even prior to first psychosis onset, during prodromal stages—and that these patterns can be used to predict eventual psychosis.

Corcoran's group interviewed thirty-four people ages fourteen to twenty-seven who had developed early symptoms of schizophrenia. During a one-hour, open-ended interview, participants described the symptoms they had experienced and the impact of these on their lives, what had been helpful or unhelpful for them, and their expectations for the future.

The paper in the journal *Schizophrenia* reported that a combination of phrase length, speech coherence, and frequency of a specific part of speech called a determiner (e.g., words like *a, this, that, both, my*) predicted the five adolescents that progressed to psychosis with an accuracy of 100 percent. Corcoran's group later tested their tool in an independent dataset from

74 UCLA and showed that, indeed, speech could be used to predict a psychotic episode with up to 82 percent accuracy.

What strikes me about Corcoran's work is that she made use of data that I already create during a standard clinical evaluation: open-ended speech. Each question I asked Irene was a probe of her behavior. Because my questions were open-ended, she could answer and guide our conversation any way she chose, allowing me to see what was on her mind. The value of an open-ended clinical conversation isn't contested, but right now, the only tool I use to evaluate it is my own brain. After my exam, I'll summarize what I've observed in my clinical note, often with one-word boilerplate descriptions. But there is much more we could do with this data.

I found it hard to engage Irene—she would reply with simple, one-word sentences and seemed poised but aloof. I noted in her mental status exam that she was "Hypoactive except, taps her right foot," but it was unclear to me what exactly this meant or how to treat this data. I was also unsure whether Irene and I had formed any therapeutic alliance—a term for the clinician-patient relationship in psychotherapy and a therapist's primary treatment instrument.

Dr. Wolfgang Tschacher is a psychologist working in Bern, Switzerland, who has spent his career trying to understand, measure, and improve therapeutic alliance. Tschacher began by using questionnaires. Following a therapy session, Tschacher would ask a patient or clinician how well they felt they got along with their therapist or how capable they felt of solving their problems. While he felt each person's experience was valid (and performed analyses showed it indeed captured part of the therapeutic alliance), he suspected he was still missing something.

There's more to the therapeutic alliance than can be captured by a questionnaire. When a patient fills out a questionnaire, Tschacher explained to me, "they can only say what they
know, what they're conscious of, aware of." Using the technologies described above, Tschacher began to measure facial
expression, movement, word choice, and voice acoustics—all
from video data that was already being produced during each
clinical interaction. He discovered that things people were
not consciously aware of—nonverbal behavior like crossing
or uncrossing one's legs, gesturing, and head nodding—were
equally important in measuring therapeutic alliance. He further learned that how much a clinician and patient's nonverbal
behavior was *synchronized* reflected the quality and outcome of
their therapeutic relationship.

A patient's nonverbal behavior was, Tschacher came to
realize, an *embodiment* of emotion, a physical manifestation
of someone's depression or someone's schizophrenia. Much
in the same way we measure heart rate with a pulse oximeter
on the finger, Tschacher argues we can measure the brain by
tracing physical movement during a normal conversation. As
I described in the Introduction, I had intuitively picked up on
the embodiment of depression or schizophrenia as I sat silently
in Dr. Wei's clinic in China. In Irene's clinical note, I had again
intuitively noted the embodiment of Irene's psychosis when I
noted "hypoactive," but this was far from a useful measure—
would the next clinician look at the word "hypoactive" and be
able to tell whether Irene was more or less "hypoactive" than
when I saw her?

If the conversation is the foundation of the psychiatric
exam, a behavioral probe for brain function, we should use

76   instruments to measure and capture it as rigorously as possible. After all, if I were evaluating any other organ—a heart, a liver, a kidney—I would use an instrument designed to help me sense what that organ is doing with greater precision, to help me measure and plot what might be a clinically useful signal. In Irene's case, this would have amounted to simply video recording our conversation and processing this data. A simple, though potentially valuable, clinical overture.

Stress Tests for the Brain

During the hour or so I spoke with Irene, I used my sphygmo-manometer, EKG, and stethoscope to measure her cardiovascular system—her blood pressure, heart's electrical activity, and the *lub-dub* of her heart valves closing at different stages of her heartbeat. I took samples of her blood and urine so I could gauge how well her kidneys were functioning based on how much creatinine, sodium, and potassium I found.

I took these measures because I have an idea—or model—of what her heart and kidneys do within her body. I (and all physicians) think of Irene's heart as a pump, and if I want to assess the health of her heart, I use instruments to measure and calculate how her pump is behaving. Within my heart-as-pump model, I think of cardiovascular disease as pump failures and pipe problems; my treatments strengthen the pump and clear clogs.

The heart is, of course, much more complex than a pump. But my heart-as-pump model is useful. The model guides me to collect specific types of data and allows me to make sense of

78   data, detect disease, and observe how and whether my treatments are bringing her pump function back to health. The model
allows me to act in such a way that I'm useful to my patient.

No one really knows how to view the brain. We also don't
really know how to measure or calculate how well the brain is
working, or how to connect the symptoms we see in mental
illness with a particular brain dysfunction. When I evaluated Irene, I observed her walking and talking, I noted how she
dressed herself (and the fact that she *was* dressed), and, in a very
commonsense way, intuited that her brain was functioning on
at least these levels. But I lacked an instrument to auscultate
Irene's brain in the way I would her heart; instead, I probed and
prodded her brain through conversation.

I've shown in the first three chapters how I met Irene as a
complete stranger and, in about twenty minutes, tried to deduce
her behavioral baseline. This isn't ideal for many reasons, not
least of which is that our encounter took place in a psychiatric
hospital when she wasn't at her baseline.

In Chapters One and Two, I presented digital tools that
could help sketch Irene's behavioral baseline. In Chapter Three,
I described tools that could help me auscultate Irene's behavior
during our interview. This would be comparable to a cardiologist measuring blood pressure—not with their eyes or fingers, but with a clinical instrument designed for that purpose.
There's an additional tool that physicians use to coax an organ
to reveal a particular deficit: stress tests.

The purpose of a stress test is to identify a problem that,
under normal circumstances, would remain invisible. To perform
a stress test, clinicians slowly ramp up an organ's function and
see where and whether that function breaks down when flexed.

In an exercise stress test, you walk on a treadmill that slowly speeds up, making your heart work progressively harder. Meanwhile, an EKG monitors your heart's electrical rhythm, a sphygmomanometer measures your blood pressure, and a pulse oximeter measures your heart rate and how much oxygen is in your blood.

The goal of the exercise stress test is to flex your heart's function and precisely detect where you might have a problem (the EKG shows where the heart's electricity is abnormal). Precision is important because the potential treatments (stents, bypass surgery) are precise. To figure out where and how the pump is broken, we stress and measure the pump.

Psychiatrists treat the clinical interview as a stress test. The moment I walked into the exam room, I began to flex Irene's brain. Later in our admission interview, I asked Irene a standard set of questions as part of my mental status exam: "Where are we right now? What's today's date?" These questions showed me that—in rough strokes—specific functions of Irene's brain were "online."

I then dug a little deeper and asked her to name the last five presidents of the U.S.A.—a rough test of memory. "Can you tell me what the phrase 'Live by the gun, die by the gun' means?" A test for abstract thinking. "Can you spell WORLD backward?" A rough test of executive function. It's useful to think of each of these questions as a type of stress test; a verbal behavioral probe, a mental treadmill that I put Irene's brain through.

But, unlike an exercise stress test, my questions don't help me understand Irene's problem with any useful precision. For example: If Irene's EKG showed an amplified waveform in the V4 and V5 leads, I understand that her left ventricle has a problem.

80   But if Irene can't spell D-L-R-O-W, I know nothing about which part of her brain (if it's indeed her brain) has a problem. My mental status exam tells me nothing specific, meaning that Irene's answers don't direct me toward a specific problem or treatment. My mental exam tells me as much about Irene's brain as asking her to do a jumping jack would tell me about her heart.

Stressing the brain is no small problem, primarily because we don't know how to think about the brain. It's not obvious. Should we think about the brain as a floating iceberg with an enormous id lurking below the water's surface? A computer? A face-recognizing machine? A chair-building machine?

There are many possible models for the brain. But what I need is a way to think about the brain that helps me design tests to flex the brain's capacity, identify a possible abnormality, and guide my treatment. My psychiatric exam was based on my clinical instincts. I need clinical tests to help me understand where, more precisely, Irene's behavior is off. In addition, I need a model of the brain that can absorb and bake in new information, the way my brain did as I interviewed Irene (more on this in Chapter Five). For this chapter, I'll view the brain as an inference machine.*

---

* As opposed to the twentieth-century idea that the brain is a "reflex machine" or even the twenty-first-century idea that the brain is a "sampling machine" that builds up an understanding of the environment by sampling the world, I use the term "inference machine" without specifying what the formal mechanism of inference is—whether active inference or reinforcement learning or other type of learning mechanism. My goal is to present a generalist argument in the hopes that I can strategically sidestep much of the (heated) debate over which mechanism the brain uses in its inference.

The Brain as an Inference Machine

The brain's most fundamental quality is that it tries to make sense of the world. The brain, many scientists argue, is an inference machine whose goal is to *actively guess* what is present in the environment and to compare these guesses to what we see, hear, and feel.

To understand why inference is necessary, consider that we are never fully in touch with our environment. Our brain is surrounded by a half-inch wall on all sides, completely sealed off from direct contact with the outside world. Our brain by itself doesn't see, hear, or feel *anything*. Instead, our brain infers what's going on based on small, incomplete signals it receives from outside its bony vault. Our sensory receptors *transduce* the environment's energy (touch and sound are pressure; light and temperature are electromagnetic energy) and pass these neural signals through our skull, to our brain.

It's difficult to describe how limited our senses are. Our eyes, for example, detect only a very narrow spectrum of light (the "visible spectrum" or 400–700 nanometers in wavelength). Yet the retina alone sends the brain a massive 1.25 GB of data each second, or twice as much as my Wi-Fi. This data is not a "video" of the world, but rather just raw, barely processed signals. Our brain has access to a sliver of the larger universe, and even this sliver represents a deluge of raw pixels and sound bites. To make matters worse, our survival often depends on us (in real time) making enough sense of this raw data to navigate an uncertain and potentially hostile terrain.

If we think of the brain as an inference machine, our brain uses sensory data to generate hypotheses or guesses about what's in the environment. A tree obviously can't pass through our skull and "exist" in our brains. Instead, our brain guesses what sensory signals it expects to receive if we are standing in front of a tree and then compares what signals it actually receives from the retina with that expectation. The closer the two line up, the more strongly we suspect we are indeed standing in front of a tree.

Imagine a forest. You're probably not thinking of a specific forest, but your mental model of what a forest ought to look like and what sort of things you might expect to be in a forest. Within your "forest" model is the expectation that you'll perceive trees (something for which you also have a mental model). Say now you're tromping through this forest. Your brain expects to receive signals from your retina that look like tree trunks: a stationary, vertical stack of brown pixels.

Because you're tromping through a forest, should you sense a stack of brown pixels in a vertical pattern, your brain would infer that there was a "tree trunk" and use this inference to avoid an unpleasant collision. (Of note, right now, I'm sitting in a Subaru dealership. I look up from my computer and my brain detects a vertical stack of brown pixels. I do not perceive this as a tree, but instead as a tree-looking brochure rack that has been emptied as a pandemic precaution. The outdoorsy brochure rack fits into my "Subaru dealership" model, but might be somewhat surprising in a forest.)

Experience has taught you that your "forest" model is very reliable, that you are so likely to perceive "tree trunk" while tromping in a forest-scenario that you probably don't even notice the trees, perceiving them subconsciously without thinking, "That's a tree . . . over there's a tree . . ." This "tree in

forest" model frees up your brain to talk to your hiking buddy or
to ruminate over your day.

But what if, after you pass a "trunk," you sense a rustling, then a growl. Then those stationary brown pixels begin to lean slightly toward you. Surprised, you look closer and notice a large shadow moving your way. Uh-oh.

Surprises are bad. A surprise means that your "trunks in forest" model failed to represent and predict reality. It means that you are tailspinning toward a state of disorder and possibly death. To minimize surprise, your brain must change something.* You can update the perception ("Oh, that's a bear!") or change the sensory data through action ("Get away from that bear-looking thing!")—in this case, you would probably do both. Either way, you have learned how to behave based on your inferences of what's in the world around you.

This is a simple story: We need to understand what's going on in the world to be able to act within it. Our brain generates models that help us anticipate what to expect in a particular environment. When our sensations align with our expectations, we are able to infer what's in the environment. When our

---

* I should note that the assumption that the brain is in the "minimizing surprise business" is specific to Karl Friston's (whom you'll meet in Chapter Five) active inference scheme; adjustments to an active inference model are motivated by the brain's assumed desire to minimize the amount of surprise, or error signal, it has with the environment. Active inference is a flavor of more general Bayesian learning theory. A different flavor of Bayesian theory is reinforcement learning, wherein correct representations of the environment are motivated by the agent's desire to maximize reward: If you correctly predict and understand an environment, you can most ably exploit that environment, maximizing the amount of benefit or reward you gain from that environment.

84 sensations and expectations are not aligned, we learn and act. We act to minimize the gulf between our sensations and expectations, learning a better model that's more fit for our environment. Why? Because errors lead toward a state of disorder, toward dissolution and death.

Viewing the brain as an inference machine allows us to create ways to test and measure different aspects of this inference process. For example, I might flash someone a picture of a tree-looking brochure rack in the midst of a forest and then measure how surprised someone feels to see it there, how certain they are that they've actually seen a tree-looking brochure rack, and how quickly someone updates their "forest" model to include tree-looking advertisements. The Bayesian brain may not be the most *correct* way to view the brain (in the same way a heart clearly isn't just a pump), but it is proving to be a *useful* way.

As noted at the beginning, viewing the heart-as-pump model has specific uses: It allows me to think of ways to stress that pump and develop instruments to measure and calculate how well her pump is behaving. Comparably, viewing the brain-as-inference-machine has specific uses: It allows me to think of ways to stress that machine and develop instruments to measure and calculate how her machine is behaving.

Below, I use three clinical examples—schizophrenia, bipolar disorder, and anxiety—to showcase types of stress tests that might prove useful in my workup of Irene.

Schizophrenia
Schizophrenia is a severely disabling illness that warps the fabric of someone's reality, often tearing it apart. Schizophrenia is sometimes characterized by visual and auditory hallucinations

as well as sometimes by quite elaborate ideas or beliefs that a patient will doggedly adhere to even in the absence of evidence.

If we view the brain as an inference machine, we might say that in schizophrenia, the brain struggles to balance what it senses with what it expects to sense, so much so that its expectations override what is actually seen, heard, and felt. Using our forest analogy, in schizophrenia, the brain so strongly *expects* to see a tree that, even in the absence of a stack of brown pixels, it perceives a tree. This is the quintessential false positive that psychiatrists call a hallucination.

A study recently published in *Science* described a type of stress test that might help us measure these doggedly stubborn models that—if we view the brain as an inference machine— underlie hallucinations. The project was led by Yale psychiatrist Dr. Al Powers in collaboration with Drs. Phil Corlett and Chris Mathys. The goal of the stress test was to try to train someone to hallucinate and then to measure what happened when they did.

In their stress test, they repeatedly showed people a checkerboard paired with a tone. Every time someone heard a tone, they'd press a button; so checkerboard, tone, button; checkerboard, tone, button. After training people on this "checkerboard then tone" model, Powers stopped playing the tone after the checkerboard. They wanted to see how different individuals would respond: checkerboard, tone, button; checkerboard, [*silence*], button?

As expected, healthy participants made a few mistakes; even a healthy mind is imperfect. But Powers discovered that people who, even before the stress test, experienced auditory hallucinations (as part of a psychosis or as self-described "clairaudient psychics") were five times more likely to "hear"

86   nonexistent tones than healthy participants. They were also more *certain* they heard nonexistent tones.

Powers had found a way to flex the brain so he could measure how someone interacts with the environment. The test further allowed him to find where in the brain a problem might be: As a participant's certainty that they heard a nonexistent tone increased, so, too, did the activity in brain regions associated with auditory perception. By devising a stress test to create a percept in the absence of sensation, Powers had found a brain region responsible for auditory hallucinations. Since publishing their work, Powers and colleagues have developed an online version of their stress test and are testing whether it proves helpful in treating patients with schizophrenia.

Bipolar Disorder

Mood, scientists think, differs from emotion: Emotions are tied to an individual event (e.g., my morning cappuccino makes me happy), while mood reflects the cumulative impact of multiple events (e.g., I was in a bad mood after I woke up late, couldn't find my keys, and then had a flat tire). Creating a stress test for mood has proven difficult.

Mood-induction tasks have historically taken the form of asking someone to watch a movie or view a series of pictures and then asking them how they feel afterward. Though such mood-induction tasks do, indeed, induce a specific mood (depending on the type of movie or picture), it is difficult to *measure* how much mood is changing moment-to-moment because it's difficult to define how a scene in a larger movie alters mood in real time.

Another way of inducing mood is with a reward task, wherein someone pulls a slot machine lever and receives (with some unknown probability) either a monetary reward or penalty and then they're asked how their mood is. The reward task allows us to *measure*: We know how much someone's reward and mood changes and can measure how these interact over time. You might imagine that if someone pulls the lever and receives $150 four times in a row, this might put them in a better mood than if they *lose* $150 with each pull. Experimental evidence in a group of nearly twenty thousand people shows this is indeed the case.

If we view the brain as an inference machine, a change in mood following a series of $150 rewards suggests that you have *learned* from your environment to be in a better mood. Flexing this connection between mood and environment and learning suggests a stress test.

By varying the amount of reward (or penalty) from trial to trial, researchers can measure how much your choices change as an indication that you have learned. For example, if you are more willing to pull the lever after winning $150 four times in a row than you are after losing $150 four times in a row, researchers can measure this change in behavior. In addition, researchers can further ask you what you think might happen in the future, or what you expect to win or lose with your next lever pull. Studies have shown that your expected outcome (i.e., how much money you anticipate winning) affects your mood as much as the actual outcome (i.e., how much money you actually win). This key measure—the difference between your expected and obtained outcomes—is called *prediction error*. The greater the error, the more you learn and update your mood.

Positive surprises (e.g., winning $150 on a single lever pull) can set you on a path toward an elevated mood. In most people, mood is fairly stable; individual rewards do not cause large shifts in mood (recall the difference between emotion and mood). But what if the seedling of an elevated mood *biases* how you perceive subsequent rewards? So much so that you have more positive prediction errors because you now perceive the actual outcome as being much higher than it actually is. Such a large gap between your expectations and reality would set you up for a big surprise, which would in turn result in an inappropriately large amount of learning.

Yael Niv and Eran Eldar, neuroscientists at Princeton and Hebrew University of Jerusalem, respectively, have conceptualized the way unexpected outcomes crescendo into a positive mood as an escalatory cycle wherein mood and perceived reward increase one another. The effect of mood on expectations is called a "mood bias," and abnormalities in mood bias are what some researchers believe might lead to bipolar disorder. You might imagine that someone with a positive mood bias is more likely to ratchet upward into a manic-like mood after winning $150 multiple times. On the other hand, you might imagine that someone with a negative mood bias might spiral downward into a depression-like mood after losing $150 multiple times.

What is useful about this stress test is that researchers and (perhaps someday) clinicians might be able to experimentally measure how a patient's learning rate and reward prediction error (surprise) change over time. Such a measure might be used to understand whether a patient is responding to treatment or whether that treatment needs adjusting.

Anxiety Disorders

Anxiety is extremely common. People with any psychiatric diagnosis are more likely to be anxious than a healthy person. Knowing that someone has a specific symptom (like having a panic attack when deciding which train ticket to purchase) is clinically useful because it suggests a treatment goal (book tickets without panicking), something to target with clinical interventions like cognitive behavioral therapy (CBT).

CBT helps patients learn to look at anxiety-provoking situations in a new, less threatening way. That you can successfully treat anxiety with CBT indicates that CBT is helpful. But on a more fundamental level, it also indicates that patients can learn how to not be anxious. If we view the brain as an inference machine, we can think of ways to dissect this learning process and understand it more precisely. We can create a stress test for anxiety.

Measuring how we learn is complex. A group of neuroscientists at Oxford University developed a reward game (similar to the reward task, above) wherein participants tried to win a pot of money. To get this money, they had to click on a green or blue rectangle, which would inch them closer (or not) to that money. Because it was unclear which rectangle (blue or green) they needed to choose, players learned which was more likely to lead to a reward by trial and error, while playing the game.

Unbeknownst to the participants, there were two versions of the game: a stable version where blue rectangles led to a reward 75 percent of the time and a volatile version wherein the reward sometimes followed blue, sometimes green. Everyone played both versions of the game, allowing experimenters to measure how quickly they could learn each version.

90   To win, people would have to mentally model how volatile the game was at any point in time. The goal of the experiment is to measure how your brain stacks up to an "ideal learner," or a computer trained to make the winning decision at every step. That seemed like a lot of computational heavy lifting.

Yet—quite surprisingly—people performed quite well, on par with the ideal learner. The Oxfordians also discovered that people played the game differently, depending on how volatile the task was. As the game switched from the steady, 75 percent version to the more volatile version, healthy people adjusted their learning rate as if it were a carefully calibrated inference machine.

To apply this stress test to anxiety disorders, a group of researchers led by Michael Browning modified this reward game— instead of winning money for choosing the correct rectangle, you'd get an electric zap if you choose incorrectly. To see how volatility affected learning rate, Browning occasionally changed the likelihood of getting shocked. Browning called this an "aversive learning task" and used it to measure how people with varying levels of anxiety navigate unsavory situations.

Browning discovered that, like the original study, nonanxious people could sense when the game was more volatile and adapt their strategy like an "ideal learner"—the more stable the task, the less an unexpected zap affected their beliefs about future events. But the more anxious a person was, the less they recognized and adapted their learning rate during the volatile game. By creating a stressful, volatile environment, Browning saw that anxious people were unable to recognize and learn in the same way healthy people were.

In their *Nature Neuroscience* paper, Browning and his colleagues wondered whether being cognitively blind to volatility could make the world seem less predictable and negative outcomes less avoidable. This in turn might further reinforce someone's overall level of anxiety, creating a spiral into deepening anxiety and other mental illnesses like depression.

While Browning's study needs to be extended and replicated, the proposed relationship between volatility and learning rate has clear clinical implications. It reduces clinical focus from cognitive symptoms (such as panic attacks when booking a train ticket), to a specific, measurable process that has gone awry. And instead of treating someone's booking a train ticket (which is simply one instantiation of an underlying problem), clinicians might use this stress test to measure how well people perceive and learn in a volatile environment and how these measures change with treatment.

Back in the Clinic

The overarching goal of each of these stress tests is to provide clinicians useful data. Each of these tests might be used in combination to provide something of a behavioral assay or inference laboratory panel that, like every clinical test I order, could then guide subsequent clinical conversation. After taking a series of measurements in my office, for example, I might sit down and discuss with my patient: "Mrs. Robinson, I'm concerned about your learning rate."

Here again, it's useful to compare mental illness to heart disease. Stress tests that treat the heart as a pump (just a simple, run-of-the-mill pump!) uncontestably oversimplify this complex

92   and elegant organ. Clinicians and patients seem comfortable reducing heart disease to a pump because it's helpful. And yet, we tend to cringe when we consider our inner lives, our own emotions and mental states, through a comparable reductionist lens by distilling our conscious experience to a few measures.

Imagine that you're in my shoes. You're a psychiatrist and a patient comes to your office. She just had a panic attack during her lunch hour while trying to book a train. She's shaken and buries her face in her hands, crying, "What if I amount to nothing!" You learn her story, about a traumatic childhood that carved the cognitive ruts in her mind. You connect with her, you empathize with her, you want to help.

Now consider your next step: Do you tell her that her brain is an inference machine and ask her to sit in front of a computer and click on blue and green rectangles? Do you tell her you're going to zap her with electricity if she chooses the wrong rectangle? Or perhaps do you tell her to watch a series of checkerboard-tone-checkerboard-tones? You acknowledge— perhaps sheepishly—that you're trying to trick her brain into hallucinating a nonexistent tone. How much confidence do you have that such games would reveal something useful about your patient's distress? Isn't her problem more complex and personal?

I'd question my devotion to reductionism here, too. These games seem too abstract and too removed from the raw, clinical realities to be taken seriously.

But recall that all of medicine went through such growing pains. The connection between heart attacks, blood pressure, and cholesterol isn't obvious. The very existence of blood pressure wasn't obvious: Even though people had seen blood spurting out of people's veins for millennia, no one thought to measure blood pressure until the eighteenth century. What such measures did was to nudge clinical conversations deeper, toward underlying and often invisible data.

The value of any clinical test is that it guides clinical practice. After all, a measurement that isn't clinically useful—that doesn't tell you something actionable about how the brain's function relates to a patient's experience—is just a nifty computational trick. The hope is that viewing the brain as an inference machine and using tests designed to stress specific aspects of the inference process will prove to be clinically useful. At present, such stress tests have shown promise, but require larger investment and evaluation before reaching the clinic.

Diagnosis
Turning Data into Action

Irene's symptoms began over a year ago. Although Irene's individual "psychosis episodes" (to use her mother's apt term) would typically last only two or three weeks, it appeared that Irene's previous personality, her relationships with her friends, and her hobbies had all become clouded by a mental illness. But which one?

Psychiatric diagnosis is a messy business.* For over a century, psychiatry has struggled to make sense of human suffering. Without question, there are certain trends and themes of suffering across individual patients. Yet, as an individual, Irene's narrative seems so unique, her life history so unlike anyone else's, that the task of summarizing her experience

* To be useful, a diagnosis must be reliable, valid, and actionable. Psychiatric diagnosis is currently based on the APA's DSM-5. For an illustration of how the DSM-5 produces a diagnosis, please see my *Scientific American* article "Should Mental Disorders Have Names?" published February 19, 2019. For a historical description of the DSM's development and purpose, please see Jeffrey A. Lieberman and Ogi Ogas's book, *Shrinks: The Untold Story of Psychiatry* (Back Bay Books, 2015).

with a diagnosis—typically, a single word—is understandably fraught with complexity.

Because Irene had prolonged periods of delusions, disorganized behavior, social isolation, and uninterest in the world outside her computer, she had lost all of her friends and was nearly flunking out of high school. She had none of the symptoms of depression or mania or OCD. She had no history of trauma. She had no history of substance use. Because she had a specific pattern of symptoms described in the DSM-5 and, crucially, because these symptoms were present in the absence of clear depression, mania, or drug use, I diagnosed Irene with schizophrenia.

But consider what the phrase "Irene has schizophrenia" means. If all you know is that Irene has schizophrenia, you have no idea which specific symptoms she has. Put differently, two people might have schizophrenia but have completely different patterns of symptoms. Such ambiguity is not unique to schizophrenia: One study humorously calculated that there are 270 million unique combinations of symptoms that would meet DSM-5 criteria for PTSD and major depressive disorder.

If all you know is that Irene has schizophrenia, you also have no idea how severe her symptoms are. Even my description of "prolonged periods of delusions, disorganized behavior, social isolation, and uninterest in the world outside her computer" holds little value. If, after being in the hospital for a week, another clinician reads my admission note describing how "Irene has prolonged periods of delusions, disorganized behavior . . ." that clinician has no way of knowing whether Irene's symptoms have improved over the past week.

Schizophrenia is not schizophrenia in the way hypertension is hypertension. Because two patients with schizophrenia

96   might have completely different patterns of symptoms, the way I treat them—from cognitive therapies to medications—might completely differ. But what's also strange is that someone with major depressive disorder might receive the same treatment as someone with schizophrenia: Antipsychotic medications can improve depression and antidepressant medications can improve schizophrenia.

If a diagnosis tells me nothing about a patient (or rather, gives me a 1-in-270-million chance of accurately describing a patient) and does not suggest which treatments might prove effective for a particular patient, then why bother diagnosing at all? Billing. I had to diagnose Irene based on DSM-5 criteria so her insurance company would acknowledge that she had a clinical problem and reimburse my hospital for her admission and treatment.

So, even though I've diagnosed Irene with schizophrenia, this label gives me no guidance about how to act to treat her. You might think this is ironic, but let me assure you that it is not: The DSM-5 does not include information about or guidelines for the treatment of any disorder because that is not why it was designed.

Diagnosis should not be detached from clinical reality, an end unto itself. The process of diagnosing is meant to help a clinician and patient more clearly define a clinical problem and, once defined, create a treatment plan that resolves that problem. Psychiatry, however, has skipped ahead to diagnosis without ever clearly defining the problem.

Creating more precise and actionable diagnoses does not require reinventing the clinical interaction. The first step is clearly defining the psychiatric problem by measuring behavior

with tools that I've described in previous chapters. The second
step is finding a way to make sense of those measurements.

Clearly Defining the Problem

Every medical specialty has struggled to clearly define clinical problems, and psychiatry is no exception. I discussed this conundrum with Dr. Tom Insel, former Director of the National Institute of Mental Health (NIMH), who since leaving his directorship has become deeply entrenched in the front lines of psychiatry's Big Data revolution. Five years ago, Insel took up a post at Verily (a sister-company of Google) where he remained until launching MindStrong, a private digital psychiatry company that I'll discuss more in Chapter Six. Throughout these ventures, Insel has been trying to define the problems that psychiatrists are trying to solve. "Just as an engineer or as anyone in tech," Insel told me, "you start by *really defining* the problems in a very explicit, very quantitative, very concrete way. And then you begin to create solutions toward those problems."

The Big Data approaches I introduce in this book represent what clinicians and researchers hope will fundamentally redefine how we think about the problems that bring our patients to the clinic. I spoke with Dr. Joshua Gordon, Insel's successor and current NIMH director, who enthusiastically told me that the digital tools promise to "change our diagnostic system and redefine how we make decisions for our patients by giving us quantitative predictions about their likelihood to respond to different avenues of therapy."

Yet, such a redefinition of mental disorders requires more than "Irene has schizophrenia" or even "Irene had prolonged periods of delusions." Defining the clinical problem requires a

98   knowledge of precisely *how disorganized* Irene's behavior was, or exactly *how many* hours Irene spends alone, in front of her computer, and how this *objectively* differs (in numbers) from her behavior one, three, or six months ago.

Big Data promises to help psychiatry measure and define a patient's clinical problem in a more precise way. And yet, even a massive amount of exquisitely precise data alone cannot guide clinical action. To be proven useful, data must have meaning and must be attached to some clinical function. Questions such as: Does a given data point or pattern of data points predict that a particular treatment will be more effective? Does a change in a given data point or pattern of data points indicate something clinically relevant—that a patient should be hospitalized? That a medication should be increased? Decreased?

This is no simple matter. There are two approaches currently being pioneered to connect Big Data with clinical action: machine learning and clinical inference.

Machine Learning to the Rescue?
Machine learning (ML) algorithms are increasingly hailed as a paradigm-shifting way forward in Big Data analyses—especially in mental health research and treatment. The primary reason is the sheer amount of data an ML algorithm can manage: While my brain might be able to juggle ten or fifteen bits of data at once, an ML algorithm is limited only by a computer's storage capacity (which continues to grow).

Most ML algorithms have a similar structure: They take a large clinical dataset and try to predict a given clinical variable. In ML parlance, the algorithm takes a large group of clinical *features* and, within these features, identifies a pattern that predicts a clinical *target variable.**

Consider our example of watching someone's shadow in Central Park from Chapter Three. Measurements of how the hips move relative to the chest and shoulders and head, how quickly the legs move and even how much the legs bend at the knees and the arms bend at the elbows at each moment (or frame) as someone walks down the sidewalk are measured, vectorized, and then used as features. An ML algorithm will take these features and, across hundreds or thousands of people, identify a pattern that predicts a clinical target variable, such as which patients have a given gait abnormality (e.g., shuffling gait) or perhaps which will require a hip replacement. Such a pattern might help clinicians identify patients who will require a hip replacement five or ten years in advance, thus allowing these patients to be treated preventatively with physical therapy to extend this horizon.

It's worth noting that an ML algorithm functions much like a clinician. When I evaluated Irene, I was looking for a certain

---

* This is known as a supervised ML algorithm. There are also unsupervised ML algorithms, in which a target variable does not need to be explicitly defined by a user. Some argue that, because even so-called unsupervised algorithms require a user to specify and provide input features, all ML algorithms are fundamentally supervised. (An algorithm cannot access data you do not provide it.) For the purpose of this book, I will focus on supervised ML algorithms. But a brief application of an unsupervised ML algorithm might be gathering measurements of how people walk (gait vectors) and identifying novel groupings of common gait patterns. Such groupings might help clinicians better identify people with different forms of gait abnormalities and more rapidly (and accurately) identify people who will need a hip replacement in a way that is more precise than and perhaps even redefines how movement disorders are currently diagnosed.

100   *pattern* of symptoms (or features) that, if present, led me to the diagnosis of schizophrenia (the target variable). As soon as I saw the presence of specific symptoms accompanied by the absence of other specific symptoms, I recognized this as a pattern that the DSM-5 defines as "schizophrenia."

But the problem is that, although I was able to do this rather efficiently—after a twenty-minute conversation with Irene paired with a ten-minute conversation with her mother—my diagnosis of schizophrenia didn't meaningfully guide clinical action.

Of course, in the absence of a clear path forward, the hope is that ML will help us identify previously unseen but useful patterns within a larger amount of data than I am able to mentally juggle. And yet, the entire clinical overture is not to identify a *pattern*—i.e., to diagnose—but rather to determine what *caused* the pattern and therefore how to act to mitigate that cause with treatment. To do this requires a different toolset.

Clinical Inference

To understand how Big Data might guide future clinical practice, I visited University College London to speak with Dr. Karl Friston, a psychiatrist who has become a leader in computational neuroscience and, more recently, an artificial intelligence guru. Friston kindly invited me to give a presentation about this book at his weekly lab meeting. Following my thirty-minute presentation, Friston led a marathon two-and-a-half-hour discussion.* Our conversation focused on whether ML algorithms—which use patterns of features to predict a target

---

* I remain grateful to Anjali Bhat, Friston's graduate student, who suggested I come prepared for a marathon meeting.

variable—might be useful in making sense of the data produced in phenotyping.

"It's not a question of just taking all this glorious data and just classifying it, of being able to diagnose, basically," Friston said, rolling the idea over in his mind. "In psychiatry, being able to diagnose means nothing unless you understand the cause, unless you can explain what's happening to the patient you've diagnosed and you can interpret it in terms of pathophysiology or indeed psychopathological mechanisms."

We discussed how every field of medicine except for psychiatry performs a similar exercise: Whenever a patient reports a symptom, the physician attempts to diagnose and treat that symptom in terms of an underlying cause, or the physiology that produced that symptom. Friston argues that this process of working backward from symptom to physiology is a type of *active inference* (which for the sake of simplicity, I will call clinical inference).* Clinical inference is the process of selectively gathering evidence that supports (or opposes) what I think might have caused a patient's symptoms. Conceptually, it is the same framework I introduced in Chapter Four to explain how our brain makes sense of our environment. I'll use an example to show how this works.

Imagine that you've been having a sharp, concerning pain in your chest every time you walk up a steep flight of stairs. You come to my office and tell me what's happened. I ask you

---

* Again, I'm using "clinical inference" in the most general sense. Formally, Friston's active inference is a type of Bayesian inference. To see how Bayesian inference might be applied to Big Data, readers may consult Schwartenbeck, P., Friston, K. (2016). "Computational Phenotyping in Psychiatry: A Worked Example," *eNeuro* 3(4), ENEURO.0049-16.2016. https://dx.doi.org/10.1523/eneuro.0049-16.2016.

102   a focused series of questions that I've learned during my medical training and, based on your answers, I exclude things like anxiety, a broken rib, or heartburn. I need more information and so I order an exercise stress test (also described in Chapter Four) to help me narrow down the possible causes of your chest pain. Narrowing down what caused your chest pain allows me to appropriately treat it. This clinical overture—the judicious use of questions and tests to work backward* from symptom to cause to treatment—is possible because I have learned a series of *generative models* that explain the underlying physiologic processes that commonly cause chest pain.

If the exercise stress test, for example, shows that your EKG looks abnormal when walking at a clipping trot, then it's likely you have a narrowing in your coronary arteries. Even though I cannot physically *see* the inside of your coronary arteries, the EKG data makes me more confident that restricted blood flow through these arteries is causing your chest pain and, in response, I might send you to an interventional cardiologist to place a stent or perform bypass surgery to resolve the problem.

Clinical inference allows me to reason backward from things that I can directly observe (your report of chest pain) and, by selectively gathering additional information (an EKG), to understand things that I cannot observe (narrowing of your coronary arteries). Clinical inference further allows me to test different hypotheses about what caused your chest pain and settle on the

---

* Backward because a problematic physiologic process has caused the chest pain to emerge. So if a patient comes to the clinic reporting chest pain, a clinician does not stop at this symptom, but rather looks upstream to the source of the problem.

hypothesis that best explains the available evidence. Having data that supports one origin for your pain simultaneously makes other explanations less likely: Knowing that your coronary arteries are narrowed makes me less suspicious that a broken rib or heartburn caused your pain. At every stage in this process, the motivation remains the same. I want to understand what caused your chest pain for the sole purpose of selecting the most effective treatment. This overall strategy is fundamentally different from the way I approached my conversation with Irene.

Psychiatrists approach clinical reasoning much more like an ML algorithm: The purpose of my clinical interview was to populate a list of features. To do this, I asked Irene a slew of questions dating back to her childhood. During this conversation, I kept—as much as possible—this information in my head, hoping that a particular pattern would pop out and help me settle on my target variable, a DSM diagnosis. So, whereas in our chest pain example, my goal was to decrease the uncertainty of which physiology conspired to cause your chest pain, my goal with Irene was to identify a pattern of symptoms I recognized. Psychiatry has structured their clinical enterprise in a fundamentally different way than other fields of medicine.

Throughout medicine, clinicians trace a patient's symptom to the underlying organ and biology that has gone awry. But in psychiatry, attempts to trace a patient's symptoms back to their physiologic cause have failed. In fact, outside of neurodegenerative conditions, if a physiologic explanation for a patient's symptoms exists, that problem is definitively no longer under psychiatry's purview—so a depressed mood caused by low levels of the thyroid hormone is a concern for an endocrinologist.

Although it might appear that psychiatry defines itself by an absence of biologic explanation, millions of dollars of research, thousands of papers, and lifetimes of work have been (and are being) poured into identifying biologic origins of mental illness. And yet, notwithstanding this effort, with the exception of neurodegenerative and rare genetic conditions, there is not a single psychiatric disorder that requires the use of a biologic measure to establish a diagnosis, stage the progression of illness, guide the selection of treatment, or evaluate the impact of treatment.

Psychiatry is in a similar position to where cardiology was after Roosevelt's death (described in the Introduction). It remains unclear which data will help unravel the complexity of mental disorders and, therefore, inform novel treatments. Though there are scattered clues about what causes mental disorders, these are no more than tentative, nascent hypotheses.

And yet, following in the footsteps of the Framingham Heart Study, the hope of the Big Data approach is that by pairing the intuitions of clinicians with the carefully calibrated results from digital devices and sensors, we can make sense of a massive amount of data and prune hundreds (if not thousands or millions) of data points down to a handful of the most clinically useful. The hope is to more clearly define the clinical problem in psychiatric diseases so clinicians can better identify and treat those problems. As in the case of hypertension, cholesterol, and smoking, it was only *after* the problem was clearly defined— that is, only *after* these three risk factors were associated with the significant morbidity of heart disease—that treatments targeting each of these risks were developed and made available to patients. In fact, it was only by measuring the blood pressure of thousands and thousands of people that our concept of hypertension was clearly defined.

The types of measures described in this book—from patterns of behavior to geographic and social activity—very well could redefine the way we think about mental illness. I enjoyed discussing with Dr. Joshua Gordon (the current director of the NIMH) how, instead of treating depression, for example, a clinician might instead treat someone's digital health, as measured by an interaction of their social media posts, geolocation, call logs, and clinical interview. Thus defined, new treatments might emerge to target specific digital measures that have an impact on outcomes—just as treating hypertension has an impact on cardiovascular risk.

The approval of new treatments to target new measures of disease would require that (in the U.S.) the FDA establish digital outcomes as a target outcome measure for clinical trials. Gordon told me that, anticipating that digital mental health apps and approaches will change the way clinicians diagnose, the NIMH and the FDA are actively engaged in multiple lines of conversation about shifting diagnosis from "depression" as defined by a clinical scale or the DSM, to, say, a "low-actimetry measure"* as defined by a passive sensing app. Treatment for low-actimetry might be an antidepressant or it might be a psychotherapeutic approach specifically targeting low-actimetry. If this works and has an impact on patient outcome, the FDA would then approve an antidepressant or an actimetry-based psychotherapy for the treatment of low-actimetry.

---

* Actimetry is a combination of accelerometer and geolocation data, essentially a measure of how physically active you are. Think Fitbit.

106 **Back in the Clinic**

As part of her admission procedure, I ordered a total of 106 individual laboratory values—measures of Irene's liver, kidney, thyroid, and immune functions, certain vitamin levels, and the presence of drugs in her urine. Though these routine tests helped rule out a host of medical conditions, not one of these tests proved useful to my eventual diagnosis of schizophrenia.

Yet this put me in a strange situation: I took rigorous measurements of things that were not useful to my diagnosis, and yet never bothered to measure rigorously the symptoms that were.

Even though I diagnosed Irene with schizophrenia, I had no idea precisely *how disorganized* Irene's behavior was— something that an analysis of her social media posts or of our clinical conversation might have provided. Although I stated that Irene was delusional, looking for clandestine messages on the internet, I didn't bother to look at her browser history and see *how often* and for *how long* she visited Urban Dictionary or Spotify or the astrology pages or whether this pattern of internet use differed from her pattern six months ago. I could have measured *how many hours* Irene spent alone by seeing how often her geolocation was her room. By consulting her call and text log, I could have measured if she was indeed more isolated from her friends than she was one, three, or six months ago.

Imagine how differently my conversation with Irene and her mother might have gone. Instead of telling Irene, "I'm sorry to hear you've distanced yourself from family and friends," I could have sat with Irene in front of a computer screen and, looking at a summary of her call and text log, said something like, "Irene, I'm afraid your mother has a point: I can see here that three months ago, you texted your friends fifty times per day and then—around the same time your internet use began to climb—it looks like you texted them progressively less until you stopped texting them entirely."

This is not just a nifty thing to do with Big Data. Measuring relevant symptoms is the very nuts-and-bolts of clinical work. Without measuring Irene's clinical problem, I cannot say with confidence whether or to what extent my intervention has improved that problem.

In the same way that I'd take repeated blood pressure measurements to test whether an antihypertensive improves my patients' hypertension, the tools I describe in this book would give me the ability to sit down with Irene and, looking at the data, discuss whether a medication is having an effect. Without the data, I just don't know.*

But further, considering Irene's clinical problems from this Big Data framework, I no longer have to fret over diagnosing Irene with schizophrenia (or not), which we discussed was not an actionable part of my evaluation. What I am left with is a behavioral assay that could help guide me to different forms of treatment.

For example, social isolation is a symptom of many psychiatric diagnoses—from depression to anxiety to PTSD. It seems quite reasonable that, by quantifying social isolation, we would be better positioned to identify treatments that might help improve social contact by 25 percent or 50 percent or some such

---

* One might argue that to learn whether a medication has had a clinical effect, I might simply ask Irene or her mother. This is a fair point and is precisely the type of imprecision that plagues psychiatry. Measurements matter because medicine is complex: Ask yourself whether you're comfortable managing your cardiovascular disease based on how well you think you feel after taking Lipitor.

number. By measuring social isolation, it becomes a clinical target, one that can anchor novel therapeutic development and provide quantitative prediction for whether someone might respond to a given therapy. Finally, such a measurement would help me know whether my treatment indeed had the desired clinical action.

And yet, even before Irene begins therapy, Big Data promises to restructure the type of treatment conversation I have by including the likelihood of success. I might be able to say something like, "Medication A has shown a 30 percent improvement in social isolation in 60 percent of patients within the first two weeks of treatment. Medication B has a 50 percent improvement but takes two months. Do you have a preference?"

This is a form of conversation familiar to cancer patients— being presented with treatment options paired with hard outcome data and probability of treatment success. Yet, to allow these sorts of conversations to take place, we first have to do the analyses, which, in turn, require a large-scale data collection effort. Ironically, although psychiatrists have access to the type of data required to perform these analyses, we are not currently recording or analyzing this data. Psychiatry remains at the stage most medical specialties were in the 1800s. We describe heart rate as "rapid" instead of measuring it as 130 beats per minute as we let our valuable clinical data slip between our fingers.

Platforms
Gathering and Making Sense of Data

The purpose of every clinical interview is to create and gather data. During my conversation with Irene and her mother, I carried a clipboard with a single sheet of plain white printer paper. During medical school, I created a template to help me remember which things to ask during a psychiatric exam. Before each exam, I'd print a copy of my template and fill it out to make sure I cover the important parts. Having used (and memorized) my template for years now, I don't bother printing it out anymore. But I still jot down the clinical data where it would go on my template.

At the top of the sheet, I sketch Irene's story—how she came to be in the hospital, what acute psychiatric symptoms she has and how long she's had them. In the middle of the page, I note her past psychiatric history, whether she has used drugs, whether she has other medical conditions, and which medications she's previously tried. Toward the bottom of the paper, I note where Irene lives, how many siblings she has, whether she has a job, and how she spends her time. At the very bottom, I jot down how

Irene performed during her mental status exam and whether she reported things like headache, nausea, or shortness of breath.

Of course, the point is not to transcribe my conversation on this single sheet of paper, but instead to distill or reduce the large amount of data I create during my conversation with Irene and her mother to what might be the most clinically relevant. I use a sparse shorthand that is (I am told) unintelligible to anyone but me, but it cues my memory when I return to my workroom to write my clinical note.

What I've done on my sheet of computer paper is create a platform to organize and guide my clinical exam. My sheet of paper designates a home for specific pieces of clinical data so, should they arise during our conversation, I know where and how to organize this data. Furthermore, because I can see at-a-glance which topics we've discussed, I can identify where I should probe more and how to make sense of what might otherwise be an overwhelmingly nuanced and complex narrative.

My sheet of paper, therefore, is a tool, a platform that guides my clinical exam, which as discussed in Chapter Five, can be formalized as a data discovery procedure, an exercise in clinical inference.

Irene and her mother presented me a large amount of data: their narratives, my personal observations of their behavior, my physical exam, my discussions with my clinical staff. During my clinical training, I learned strategies to mentally organize and identify important signals within this host of clinical data. However, I should emphasize that even though I've devised a way to record bits of information on my paper platform, I am *mentally* organizing, which means that I'm relying on my brain to make sense of what I've seen and heard in real time. It is not easy.

In the preceding chapters, I've described emerging technologies that promise to dramatically expand the amount of clinical data that I need to juggle, making it impossible for me to organize this data in my mind or on my single sheet of blank white paper. Without a platform to help me organize and make sense of the data I describe in this book, that data would be useless.

In this chapter, I describe the types of platforms that will be necessary to make these technologies clinically feasible.

Digital Health Platforms

Psychiatry is in the enviable position of having access to technologies to rigorously measure what we all agree is clinically relevant data. I routinely ask my patients how much they're sleeping, how active they are, what they're thinking about; and I've described a series of tools that have been specifically designed to measure these very things. They are already being used (with astonishing levels of success) by tech companies to measure, trace, and act on our habits and patterns.

Notwithstanding the widespread implementation of digital measurements in the tech world and notwithstanding impressive studies showing how digital measures could augment healthcare, the routine application of these tools has not yet been adopted in psychiatry to measure, trace, and improve our mental health. It is tempting to view this disconnect as simply a Luddite's refusal to embrace technology, perhaps even as clinicians' stubborn refusal to admit that what we're doing might be improved. But the situation is not quite so simple.

In Chapter Two, I described how Dr. Linda Porrino developed, tested, and published a framework to include accelerometer data in the diagnosis and treatment of childhood ADHD.

112   Although Porrino published her work in 1983, at no point in my formal training to be a psychiatrist was I taught to use or interpret accelerometer data. I've never seen a clinician use accelerometer data.

I asked my colleagues why they thought this might be the case. One colleague wondered if accelerometers were too expensive (but quickly reasoned she had accelerometers in her phone and watch). Another suggested it was because no one had developed a workable user interface or sought FDA clearance to make a clinically reimbursable or billable product. Others told me that clinicians simply don't believe they need an instrument to measure something that they can either ascertain themselves or just ask a patient about.

Consider the scale: a fairly old and ubiquitous technology we use to measure body weight. You might have a scale in your home, but, without question, every primary care physician has one in their office. We all agree that body weight is a useful measure to keep track of and so, at each clinical encounter, your primary care physician measures your weight and records that number in your medical record. Measuring weight in combination with blood pressure, heart rate, and temperature—together, called "vitals"—is a standard, billable clinical procedure. For a clinician to simply ask you how much you weigh ("How's your weight?") or, perhaps slightly better, to eyeball your weight based on their clinical experience would be absurd. That's not how we do things, because why would we? Everyone has a scale, it takes at most fifteen seconds to measure weight, and crucially, there is a framework for organizing, making sense of, documenting, and billing for scale-based weight measurements. Measurements of weight have become part of our clinical ecosystem.

Clinical tools must fit within the clinical ecosystem. Although Porrino proved that her digital tool added value to a specific facet of the clinical process, the accelerometer did not enter the clinical ecosystem. There was no way to incorporate accelerometer data into an existent clinical workflow and, crucially, there was no formalized FDA clearance of or financial reimbursement for accelerometer data. Progress in digital health (or any field) requires more than an elegant research paper showing a particular type of data or analysis is useful. It requires a platform to collect, make sense of, and bill for that data.

Software platforms have two parts: a front end and a back end. The front end software is essentially an app that a patient (or research participant) downloads onto their smartphone. Patients interact with the front end software as it collects and transmits their data to a central server. From a central location, the back end software does the behind-the-scenes heavy lifting. The back end software is responsible for analyzing, securely storing, and returning the data in a useful format to the original front end app or a different front end interface like a web browser.

To learn about digital health platforms, I traveled to Boston to speak with Dr. J. P. Onnela, an associate professor of Biostatistics at Harvard University's School of Public Health. Since 2013, Onnela has led the development of Beiwe,* one of the largest research-oriented digital phenotyping platforms in

---

* Pronounced "Bee-Wee." Onnela is Finnish and Beiwe is the name of the solar deity of the Sami, an indigenous Finno-Ugric people. The name references the complex yet powerful relationship between personal experiences, physical environment, and mental health—all different aspects of the lived experiences that the Beiwe platform seeks to bridge.

114   academia.* Onnela explained five overarching design principles that sculpt the development of any digital platform: The
first three—data granularity, type, and platform interoperability—concern practical aspects of data collection, while the
final two—ownership and security—concern essential philo-
sophical and ethical questions, the answers to which I believe
will determine the success of this field.

Data granularity. Biomedical studies have notoriously low
reproducibility rates. One reason for this low reproducibility
is that different groups of scientists use different methods to
analyze their data. Reproducibility is a problem in digital health
because there are broadly two ways of collecting digital data.
One is to use proprietary software development kits released by
Apple, Google, and others, which provide a summary statistic
of the specific sensor data (e.g., an accelerometer's raw data is
summarized as a step count); the other is to collect raw data as it
is produced by the sensor.

Although summary statistics decrease the downstream
computational and storage burden, there are multiple limita-
tions. Some summary statistics are produced by proprietary
code that is unavailable to researchers, meaning that researchers
cannot access or assess how raw data is analyzed to produce a
given summary statistic. Because they cannot access the underlying code, researchers can also not determine how this code

---

* There are many digital phenotyping platforms: Brighten, developed by Dr.
Patricia Areán and colleagues at the University of Washington (with funding
from the NIH and also from private investment), or Mind Logger, developed
by Dr. Arno Klein and colleagues at the Child Mind Institute (with funding
from the NIH and also from private investment), to name two.

changes over time with, say, an updated software release from
the manufacturer. For example, the same person wearing two
identical smartwatch accelerometers might get different step
counts if each smartwatch uses different software updates.
Beyond the problem of standardizing what constitutes a "step,"
summarizing accelerometer data as "steps" represents an *a
priori* hypotheses about where a relevant signal might be and
how data should best be represented—hypotheses that might
prove unfounded or unhelpful as the field progresses. Further,
while raw accelerometer data might prove helpful in identifying
subtle abnormalities in movement (e.g., tremors or a shuffling
gait), a "step" count prevents this identification.

If a platform's front end collects and transmits raw data just
as it comes off the sensor, this raw data can then be stored and
processed entirely by the back end, thus allowing that same data
to be reanalyzed when better methods become available. It also
allows data collected from different operating systems (more
on this below), different time points, and different studies to
be pooled. Collecting raw data further allows the uncertainty
of that data to be calculated and accounted for, which, Onnela
explained, was often overlooked in digital phenotyping research.
A data point's uncertainty is how closely the reported value is to
the actual value. For example, the uncertainty of your geolocation on Google Maps is represented by how large your "dot" is on
the map: If your geolocation is accurate to within fifty meters,
the dot will be large, and if it's accurate to two meters, the dot
will be small. No instrument is perfect, so understanding an
instrument's inaccuracy is essential if you intend to use it to
guide your decisions.

Data type. There are two overall types of digital data: passive and active. Passive data (like those described in Chapters One through Three) can be gathered on digital devices someone already has without requiring them to do any additional work (they should just keep doing what they're already doing). Active data (like the stress tests described in Chapter Four) requires someone to actively engage the technology. Common examples of active data include a patient's response to clinical questionnaires (ecological momentary assessment, or EMA) or a recording of their voice or facial expression in a video diary. The limitation to active data collection is that it requires participant engagement, which may not happen over an extended period of time. People might forget, become disenchanted with the technology, or eventually just quit.* Because the overarching goal of digital health is to characterize the largest number of participants over the longest possible horizon, passive data appears to be a useful way to accomplish this by not asking users to do anything they aren't already doing.

Platform interoperability. Interoperability is a platform's ability to function on multiple operating systems, which is an essential part of a scalable digital health platform. Being able to

---

* At the beginning of my third year of residency, I enthusiastically gathered every clinical scale I could find (about forty total) into a file folder. Third year focuses on outpatient psychiatry and, during this year, I decided to ask my patients to keep track of how their symptoms changed over time by actively journaling their sleep, anxiety, or depression questionnaires between our scheduled visits. Many of my patients agreed to the exercise; only one continued for two months. They either forgot to fill out their journal, lost their journal, or simply decided they didn't want to do it. I stopped the exercise.

operate on Android and iOS allows a platform to access about 99 percent of all smartphones, and therefore reach as many people as possible. Interoperability isn't simply a matter of maximizing the number of users, but rather of maximizing the epidemiologic quality of the data.

iOS phones, Onnela explained to me, have much higher average annual incomes than Android users. Consider that, according to one analysis, Android users have an annual income of $61,000 per year while iOS users make $85,000. Although the absolute difference is only $24,000, this is nearly 40 percent more income. Interoperability allows a platform to reach as wide a socioeconomic profile as possible. Research has shown that— in addition to health outcomes—socioeconomic status moderates multiple downstream factors, such as how often someone might use a technology (known as the "cost of time" per hour for that person) and what types of services someone might use.

Ownership. Who owns what is a contentious issue in science— whether in the academy or industry. Without exception, every person I interviewed while researching this book had an opinion about data and software ownership. One of the primary reasons why large-scale, cross-platform, collaborative digital phenotyping studies have not been performed is simply because no one can agree on who will own the data. Do patients own their data? Does a health system? University? Insurance company? Tech company? Because no one can agree, each of these stakeholders is currently gathering their data within their own (relatively) small, walled garden.

The politics of data and software ownership seem aligned with individuals' stake in digital health. An academic is more likely to promote openness and data sharing because the academic business model (which is based on publication and grants) does not directly depend on data ownership. Onnela, for example, openly shares Beiwe's source code—so much so that he's designed it to allow a research group to download the platform, upload the back end onto Amazon Web Services, and, ideally, in a few hours, have a functioning digital phenotyping platform. Because Onnela does not rely on Beiwe's commercialization to continue its development (or pay his or his staff's salary), his primary goal is to decrease barriers to entry and enable as many research groups as possible to use his tool to gather data.

For an industry researcher, however, data is money. Although industry would also benefit from an expansion of data collection, most tech companies' business models are based on owning rights to data and intellectual property, both of which allow them exclusivity and therefore market share. Industry software is proprietary primarily because it provides a unique analysis or summary statistic that has commercial value.

As of now, the question of ownership in digital health has not been answered. There are multiple ongoing private-public partnerships (more below); however, there seems to be an underappreciation of the sheer amount of effort that will likely be required to make sense of digital health data. Collecting data is only a first step: Converting it into a clinically useful tool is something else entirely.

Data security and privacy regulation. Closely related to ownership is how data is secured and whether this security meets local privacy regulations. In the U.S.A., all digital health data must

meet HIPAA guidelines. In the European Union, the General Data
Protection Regulation specifies that certain kinds of patient data
can never leave the EU. This means that if a researcher wants to
run a study in Germany, that data cannot be transmitted to or
processed on a server located in the U.S.A. Therefore, researchers
collecting data in Germany must transmit, store, and process
that data on a server based in the EU.

In addition to security, privacy is an essential concern.
Here, it's not yet clear what granularity of data—raw sensor
data or summary statistics—people will be comfortable sharing
as part of their health record, primarily because it's not yet clear
what this data will tell us or how it might be exploited.* People
seem generally unconcerned about sharing their step count
with a tech company (which nearly every device with an accelerometer does), but people do seem concerned about sharing
their geolocation pattern—even though their cell service pro-
vider knows and traces where they are at all times.

I discussed this topic with Dr. Justin Baker, a psychiatrist
at Harvard University and the Scientific Director for McLean

---

* For example, some scientists are concerned that, because each person's
brain has a unique pattern of gyri and sulci, an MRI scan of a person's
brain should be considered identifiable, protected health information and,
therefore, not openly released to the public alongside that person's clinical
details. The concern is that even without clear identifiable data (such as
a name, home address, or date of birth), an unidentified individual could
technically *be* identified based on their brain's "fingerprint." To this claim,
other scientists reply that, to pair an individual and their brain MRI would
not only require the presence of two brain images (one linking the brain to
the person; the other linking the brain to the unidentifiable clinical data),
but also the creation of an enormous database with comparably enormous
computational power—which resource (barring a top-secret government
project or the efforts and financing from some evil billionaire genius/villain)
doesn't currently exist. A similar debate applies to genetic data.

120 Hospital's Institute for Technology in Psychiatry. Baker has received multiple grants to collect digital data on severely ill patients over the space of months and years—both in the hospital and at their homes. When he presents his research at conferences or public forums, he invariably gets asked what Big Data means for patient privacy—"Why do we want a Big Brother state?"

To this, Baker told me, he simply responds, "We already have one." Baker explains that our digital devices are already monitoring our mood, geolocation, and thought patterns. Right now, this monitoring occurs as part of government surveillance in the name of security, or as part of an industry-wide data collection procedure to market and sell us products. Security surveillance and marketing surveillance, as Baker calls them, already exist—it is healthcare surveillance that lags far (perhaps decades) behind. The difference between these three is that health surveillance could have practical, real-time benefits for patients.

The question really isn't so much *how* to produce data—smartphones and tech companies are already producing the data described in Chapters One and Two—but rather how to overcome concerns about ownership and security to gather enough data in one place to make sense of and incorporate useful measures into the clinical ecosystem. The underlying question facing the field is who—individual academic laboratories funded by the NIH, small startup companies, Big Tech, or governments—is best positioned to create an operable Big Data digital health ecosystem. Though the solution remains unclear, what is clear is that it'll take more than a single sheet of blank white paper.

Who Pays?

When I spoke with Dr. Joshua Gordon at NIMH, he was aware of the great possibilities that Big Data provides psychiatry to redefine clinical care. Gordon was also keenly aware of the many barriers to creating such a Big Data ecosystem.

"We need interactable solutions that are flexible," Gordon told me. He described how just accessing raw data—a key feature of a scalable, interoperable Big Data ecosystem—was a major barrier because of proprietary concerns. "How can we get the smartphone data we need, coupled with the search data, coupled with this and that in a way that ensures privacy and allows us to build the databases that we need to be able to prove things work?" Gordon asked rhetorically. Once we have access to this data, he continued, making sense of and reporting back the relevant features of the data so clinicians can use them with patients to create a treatment plan is another unresolved problem—"a huge, huge barrier."

Big Tech companies are the obvious leaders in creating a Big Data ecosystem, and yet they—understandably—keep their data and data processing algorithms proprietary: That's how they maintain their business. NIMH is getting around this technological hurdle by funding academics to build their own systems, Gordon explained, referring to emerging platforms like Beiwe, Brighten, and Mind Logger. But he also pointed out how, ironically, academics were reinventing tools already developed and maintained by Big Tech. "Why would we have to do that? Google's already got the best possible system for accumulating all this stuff, but we can't get access to their data." NIMH, Gordon argued, was not designed to function like a tech company.

122   Consider Dr. Danielle Schlosser: Five years ago, Schlosser was an assistant professor of Psychiatry at the University of California, San Francisco, where she directed a highly successful translational neuroscience laboratory that developed digital therapeutics for people with serious mental illness. She had received many highly competitive grants to fund her research, including NIMH's prestigious career development award. Before writing a subsequent grant (an R01), she was invited to present her research in person at NIMH. She nailed the presentation and was invited to apply for a special grant reserved for rising stars: a BRAINS award.

At the time, Dr. Tom Insel was NIMH director and so, before submitting her BRAINS grant, Schlosser reached out to Insel to pitch her idea for a virtual mental health clinic built around the digital therapeutics she had developed. Insel was, Schlosser told me, "thrilled about it, and he just said, 'Listen, Danielle, I really don't think you're going to be able to do that in academia.'"

Insel had recently announced that he would be leaving his NIMH directorship to take a position at Google Life Sciences (now Verily Life Sciences). Dismayed that psychiatry still defined disease based on clusters of clinical symptoms, Insel hoped that he might find a way to use some of the tools described in this book to redraw psychiatric diagnoses and advance treatment. Insel left academia's focus on grants and publication for industry's focus on product development. He invited Schlosser along, hoping she would help Verily launch her dream clinic. She accepted.

"I wanted to work with a company with resources," Schlosser told me, "and that also coupled serious science with rigor. Having someone like Tom Insel showcased [Verily's]

level of seriousness about the work. I was really impressed."
Schlosser helped Verily build OneFifteen.

OneFifteen is a tech-enabled, nonprofit recovery eco-system in Dayton, Ohio, that seeks to reduce opioid-related deaths (which, in 2017, were 115 each day across the U.S., hence the name OneFifteen). Based on a care model that combines in-person and virtual clinical visits, OneFifteen is a partnership between Verily, Kettering Health Network, and Premier Health that uses technology to improve the quality of clinical care and extend wraparound services to people in recovery from opioid abuse. After months of planning and design, the five-acre campus opened doors in October 2019. To date, it has seen over a thousand patients.

Because OneFifteen built in virtual care (such as telemedicine), when the 2020 pandemic occurred, converting to completely virtual visits was seamless and had an unexpected consequence: While the show rate across OneFifteen before the pandemic was 55 percent, Schlosser told me this skyrocketed to 85 percent. Verily's interest in OneFifteen is to improve patient care. "Verily has invested in measurement capabilities since day one," Schlosser told me as we discussed the types of digital tools in this book. Having already invested in a glucose-sensing device and software for diabetic patients, Verily anticipates applying the same principles to mental health care.

What I find encouraging about OneFifteen is that it represents a hybrid of the traditional brick-and-mortar clinic and cutting-edge technology. Without dismantling the classic patient-physician relationship, Schlosser described ways that Verily had made that interaction more fulfilling and useful—it reminded me of the difference between handwritten letters

124   and email. Every patient at OneFifteen is informed that Verily
is collecting data to improve their care and, before entering,
consents to this process—again, comparable to the way Google
uses email data to improve Gmail.

Schlosser told me that her team recently developed a
"quality metrics dashboard" and that they're figuring out how
to present the data they collect in a meaningful way to clinicians and patients. They hope to gather data about how people
recover from opioid use and what they can do to promote better
outcomes. Her goal is to use data to have discussions with
patients, helping them realize, "Okay. So if I do X, Y, and Z, I have
an 80 percent likelihood of doing well. I'm going to do that." But
before you have the results, you have to collect the data.

Partnerships between health networks and tech companies,
Insel told me, are becoming increasingly more common. Health
networks or insurance companies are interested in reducing
costs, which are primarily amassed by emergency room visits
or inpatient hospital stays. So, if a research group or tech company has developed a tool they think might improve health outcomes, help clinicians better treat patients, or otherwise help
keep people healthy outside the hospital, this is a product that
would interest a hospital system or an insurance company.

Despite the vast amount of research funding that goes into
mental health, very few products have emerged from academia.
As Insel is someone who left a highly successful academic career
as director of NIMH to become a leader in the private world, I
asked him why he thought this was the case. "In mental health,
more than most other areas," Insel told me, "there's a fairly deep
chasm between the academic world, which is about publishing

and promotion, and the world of healthcare, which is about costs   125
and outcomes, and really driven, on the tech side, by products."

Insel described how some of this chasm can be explained by
the approach the U.S. has to healthcare, generally. Single-payer
systems like in the UK and Australia have succeeded much better
in spanning this chasm, and technology has made much greater
inroads to mental health care. "But in the United States, it's
unfortunate, but healthcare is first and foremost a business here,
not a service. And it's certainly not a right. And that business is
less interested in rigor and managed care than managed costs."

Back in the Clinic

Imagine how my visit with Irene and her mother might have
been different with the tools I've described in this book. Before
I met with Irene, she and her mother might have sat down with
a "Digital Navigator," who described which types of data we felt
might be useful for us to look at together. If Irene consented,
my staff would have gathered, analyzed, and created useful measures of Irene's baseline. Then, when we spoke, our clinical conversation would have been recorded and analyzed—not simply
on my single sheet of white paper, but using state-of-the-art
tools to understand how Irene was constructing sentences, how
her facial expression changed during our conversation, how well
our nonverbal behavior was synchronized. After our conversation, I might have ordered a series of stress tests to better tease
apart which facets of how she interacts with her environment
were awry and how I might best intervene.

All of these measures would be gathered and presented
into a common platform. Throughout Irene's admission, her

clinicians would meet with her daily to see how she was progressing, to trace how she responded to the different medications or therapies Irene received in the hospital.

But an obvious and critical part of Irene's mental health care is what happens after she's discharged from the hospital. In the traditional, brick-and-mortar approach to mental health care, when Irene is ready to go home, her clinical team would schedule a follow-up appointment with (in Irene's case) a new outpatient clinician. Let's say I'd never met Irene before and they scheduled an appointment with me: "We've scheduled your appointment for later this week with Dr. Barron," the clinical team might tell Irene, handing her my contact information and our appointment date and time printed out on a piece of paper.

If I was her new outpatient clinician, her hospital team might send me a typed-up hospital summary that contains a brief description of why she came to the hospital, what happened while she was there, and the treatment plan they organized before she left. But that's all the information I'd have about Irene. Irene would still enter my office as a complete stranger—if she enters at all.

"Lost to follow-up" is a common clinical euphemism for "we have no idea what became of this patient." Studies have shown that anywhere from 30 to 80 percent of patients do not remain in mental health treatment after they leave the hospital.* Patient attrition underscores a fundamental problem with the brick-and-mortar model of care: I only know a patient is doing well if they contact *me*, meaning if they show up for

---

* Yes, that's a very wide range. Between the lines, I interpret this as meaning, "We know some come back and some don't."

their next appointment, or call or email me. When we consider app-based therapies, passive behavioral measures, and the possibility to digitally interact with patients after they leave, the attrition equation becomes much more favorable. But the question remains: How could I get Irene to interact with my clinic's app or therapy once she leaves the hospital?

As described above, the problem of implementation—not simply for clinicians and policymakers but, perhaps more importantly, for patients—is highly complex. In the same way a medication is useless if a patient doesn't take it, even if a platform seamlessly incorporates digital health data into the clinical ecosystem, that platform is completely useless if patients don't engage it. There are many obstacles to patient engagement. One study reported the grim statistic that over half of people who download a mental health app uninstall it within the first two weeks. And, of course, for an app to collect passive data, the participant has to carry their phone with them and keep it charged.

Dr. Patricia Areán is a professor of Psychiatry and Behavioral Sciences at the University of Washington. As a licensed clinical psychologist and a digital health implementation scientist for over twenty years, Areán's research has had a dual-pronged approach: figure out what's effective and figure out how to get people to do it.

In a recent study published in *JAMA Network Open*, Areán and colleagues described the counterintuitive observation that the most highly downloaded health apps aren't necessarily the most used. They evaluated apps available on Apple and Android devices with more than ten thousand downloads and saw how many monthly subscribers each app reported. To do this, they created a new metric: "stickiness." Stickiness is the measure of how many active users an app has divided by the total number of downloads. A "sticky" app is one that has many monthly users *and* downloads, whereas an "unsticky" app might have many downloads but can't seem to retain monthly users.

Areán's group found that all of the ten most downloaded apps and nine of the top ten "stickiest" apps were from private developers (i.e., not made by academics). They also noticed that "sticky" apps tended to have specific functions: Some focused on meditation, some on cognitive training or targeted alcohol or cigarette use. There wasn't a "sticky" all-in-one app, but people preferred apps for specific tasks—much the way we use apps now.

When I spoke with Areán about her work, she described how the two hot spots for user drop-off are right after they sign up and then four weeks after treatment. People tend to uninstall or stop using an app for reasons that aren't fully clear—something that in a brick-and-mortar model would be considered treatment failure or attrition. "But you shouldn't expect app engagement to be what you see in mental health," she insisted. "Some people use an app because they have an immediate need and when that need is resolved, they might turn to a different app, but they're not using yours." If the same need arises again, she explained, the user might circle back to your app.

I mentioned how I use Google Maps and Waze—both navigation apps—but for different reasons. If I just want to get somewhere, I'll use Google Maps, but if I want to see why the traffic is slow, know where there are cops giving tickets, or have

Cookie Monster shout out my directions,* I'll use Waze. Even within the same category, each app has different strengths that drive users to them. Mental health apps, Areán showed, are no different.

So perhaps Irene wouldn't be asked to download *one* app for all of her mental health care, but instead a handful of apps, each designed with a specific function in mind. And, because Irene is particularly skilled with technology (especially with web browsing), it seems possible that she might be "prescribed" a different combination of apps from another patient who has lower technologic literacy.

Just as with any medication, perhaps apps could be prescribed not simply based on which functions they offer, but also on the likelihood that the patient would actually engage and, therefore, benefit from them. And similarly, just as a patient begins to take their outpatient medication while still in the hospital, it seems plausible that Irene, before she returns home, would begin to engage her prescribed apps so she could discuss how and whether she wants to use them with her treatment team. After she leaves the hospital, Irene's handful of apps might then have a cumulative effect similar to a combination of medications—except in this case, they would provide an outpatient clinician a way to digitally check in with Irene to make sure those same treatments were helping her return to her baseline.

Of course, all of this is futurescoping. None of the tools I've described currently exist in a clinically ready form. But I've

---

* Waze's Cookie Monster function is perhaps the single most important contribution of any tech company to road trip navigation that involves toddlers. In June 2020, our trip from Connecticut to Washington was entirely guided by Cookie Monster.

130 tried to describe what I find promising and why I am excited about them alongside possible obstacles. The overarching concern with platforms is who will pay for them and how the data will be organized, secured, and distributed. There are no clear answers to these questions right now. But it is clear that it will require a large, collaborative investment of capital and time.

Conclusion

I am sitting at Yale's Saint Raphael Hospital at the height of the 2020 pandemic.* I'm a fourth-year resident but, today, am functioning as an attending; the attending-of-record hasn't left his home for two weeks because he's over sixty-five years old and at high risk for COVID. A kind man that I know well and respect, he, comfortingly, reminded me, "You're pretty much an attending anyway. You've got this." This morning, I rounded on ten patients and consulted the medical floor about a suicidal patient. It's the eleventh of April 2020. The day before Easter.

The research I did for this book—my site visits, conversations, and presentations over the last eight months—seems so

---

* Going through my final edits on December 19, 2020, I realize that this sentence, written what seems like a decade ago, was overly optimistic in a naïve and hopeful and self-soothing way. April 2020 was only the peak of the *first wave* of the pandemic. The pandemic is, of course, ongoing with no clear end in sight. I read this morning that the virus mutated and London is on lockdown. Although these paragraphs represents disproven hopes, I will leave them untouched as an example that even though I wrote this book in hopes that these tools will prove helpful, hopes can often be misleading or simply wrong.

132   long ago, from a distant world. The last month has seen an explo-
        sion in telemedicine. Telemedicine has existed for over thirty
        years, long enough for certain states to legislate for and against
        it. Many of the digital tools I've described in this book have been
        available for at least a decade. Porrino's study of accelerome-
        ters in childhood ADHD is from 1983. Google first used search
        records to trace flu outbreaks in 2008. De Choudhury used Face-
        book posts to predict post-partum depression in 2013.

        I began this book with the working assumption that I'd be
        hard-pressed to convince my patients to sign up for the menu
        of technologies I describe in these pages. And yet, the pandemic
        has disproven that assumption. People embraced geolocation
        data as a way to measure the efficacy of social-distancing efforts
        and to trace the spread of COVID-19. People with digital ther-
        mometers are uploading their temperature data to online data-
        bases, helping our health officials track outbreaks of the virus in
        real time. Google is showing how search data—this time for "I
        can't smell"—is a powerful epidemiologic tool that correlates
        almost perfectly with positive coronavirus tests and can predict
        brewing hot spots. We are pulling together and using every-
        thing, anything in our power, to fight this virus.

        I was wrong. People have *already* embraced the digital tech-
        nologies I describe here. That's why there are more smartphones
        than people on the planet. That's why Amazon and Google and
        Facebook can market products and ideas to us so well: We have
        already left behind our digital breadcrumb trail, one that Big
        Tech companies already follow and gobble up. People by and
        large are hungry for and willing to accept and interact with tech-
        nologies that improve their lives. It is we, the medical experts

and the mental health industry, that lag behind and have not yet
channeled these digital technologies into useful clinical tools.

Curious Quibbles of the Luddite Kind

Whenever a new technology emerges, it's easy to mentally bin
it into a dichotomy: Is it useful or not? Technologies are rarely
"useful or not" or "good or bad," but rather useful in certain circumstances, under certain conditions.

For example, I had a delightful conversation with an older
colleague and mentor at Yale who warned me (with the greatest
sincerity) that digital measures might be terribly misleading:
"What if you look at a given patient's face expression data
and, because the computer tells you it's normal, discharge that
patient and they commit suicide?"

I reminded him that no single tool was intended to be used
in isolation, in the same way that no single clinical test was
intended to be used in isolation. If someone has a heart attack
minutes after a normal EKG, we don't throw our hands up and
stop doing EKGs. We instead take a repeat measurement or look
to another tool (like a troponin or echocardiogram) to help us
understand what happened and how to act.

Along the same lines, imperfection should not be equated
with failure. The first week of April 2020, I had a Zoom conversation with Dr. Onnela, the associate professor at Harvard University who developed Beiwe (you met him in Chapter
Five). We both spoke from home offices and were intermittently
interrupted by our energetic toddlers. Onnela told me how a
colleague, when reviewing his paper on the quality of Beiwe's
GPS location data, commented that Beiwe had only succeeded

134   in collecting 50 percent—a mere half!—of the data available. "How valuable is this data if we're only getting half?" the reviewer bemoaned.

Onnela told me how he responded to the reviewer by writing, "Yes, we're only gathering 45,000 locations per person per day whereas we should be getting 90,000. In that sense, it's only working half as well as it could be."

"That's 45,000 locations? Each day?" I said with a deep laugh that made my microphone crackle. (Reviewers of academic journals are famous for shortsighted comments.)

"Yes," Onnela replied. "There's diminishing returns to getting a thousand pings a day to ten thousand to a million." People are quick to try to identify problems with any new technology.

I pointed out that 45,000 is far more accurate than 0, which is how many data points I had when Irene walked through my door. Furthermore, for many of the forms of data that I describe in the book, there aren't currently any measurements—not simply bad measurements, but literally none. I find it difficult to understand why someone would dismiss 45,000 measurements because it's not 90,000.

Psychiatric Care as a Service
Just before the pandemic in early March, I met with Justin Baker of the Institute for Technology in Psychiatry. I asked Baker why digital analytics hadn't been adopted full-force in medicine and, in particular, in psychiatry.

He made the point that clinicians practice the way they were trained in residency, so convincing clinicians to adopt new ideas or tools is extremely complex (and unlikely). Although he had successfully leveraged goodwill among his McLean colleagues to conduct several research studies, like Schlosser (see Chapter Six), he had begun to wonder if he could collect the type of data needed as an academic. To test the waters of industry, Baker had recently begun working part-time with Verily as a mental health expert and was surprised by how nimble the organization is.

Baker felt that, based on his experience with large health systems, digital phenotyping was likely to enter psychiatry not through academia, but through simple market demand capitalism. We discussed whether a private company might provide an online, fee-for-service product that offers digital evaluations of mood or thought or social behavior (or something). Based on this evaluation, the company might connect individual patients with a specific type of treatment or clinic.

Mental health care is notoriously underfunded. Insel told me that mental health care was, on average, only 2.4 percent of an insurance company's overall expense, which seems about right: SAMHSA reported that mental health spending was only 5.5 percent of overall healthcare expenses in the U.S. And yet it's clear that quality mental health care is something that people want and will pay a great deal of money for. Measure-based care could very well be the ultimate form of healthcare capitalism: a position where the interests of companies and patients are aligned to produce the best outcome.

All of this is far in the future, but not that far. I guess we'll see.

I wish to thank Irene and her mother for allowing me to use their story to show how I think my evaluation and treatment could be improved with technology. I also wish to thank Nicholas Lemann and Jimmy So for the opportunity to write this book and for their helpful editorial direction and encouragement. Also thanks to Camille McDuffie and Elise Caraveo for keeping me financially afloat as I flew, trained, ferried, and drove to meet with the people you met in this book.

Another thank-you to Michael Lemonick and Claudia Wallis, who both launched me on this path by teaching me how to write a good story both by example and by editing my not-so-good stories.

I presented the concepts described in this book to my colleagues at Yale University, at Harvard's School of Public Health and Center for Brain Circuit Therapeutics, at the Wellcome Trust Centre for Neuroimaging at University College London, at the Nathan Kline Institute, at the University of Washington's Center of Excellence in Neurobiology of Addiction, Pain, and Emotion, and at IBM's Computational Psychiatry and Neuroimaging division. I am grateful to my mentors at Yale, John Krystal and Todd Constable, for their encouragement to write this book and for their helpful insights. I remain grateful to Peter Fox who, as my friend and dissertation advisor, introduced me to experimental medicine and otherwise encouraged me to think quantitatively. I am also grateful to the many people of varied expertise for engaging conversations that made researching this book a delight, including: Abigail Greene, Adrian Bonenberger, Albert Powers, Alexandra Hopkins, Arno Klein, Brett Stacey,

138   Carl Zimmer, Charles Chavkin, Cheryl Corcoran, Cindy Lin, Corey Horien, Danilo Bzdok, Daniel Levy, Daniel Reiznik, Danielle Schlosser, Dave Nussbaum, Dave O'Connor, David Tauben, Dustin Scheinost, Eran Eldar, Eugene Duff, Evelyn Lake, Guillermo Cecchi, Habib Rahimi, Howard Zonana, Joe Taylor, Jonathan Rossier, Joseph Fridman, Josh Gordon, JP Onella, Justin Baker, Karl Friston, Kelsey Quick, Kely Norel, Liam Mason, Lindsay Hanford, Lisa Fucito, Lisa Messeri, Matthew Nour, Mehraveh Salehi, Menachem Fromer, Mia Handler, Michael Browning, Michael Bruchas, Michael Fox, Michael Mitoussus, Mike Milham, Munmun De Choudhury, Patricia Areán, Patrick Schwartenbeck, Peter Dayan, Peter Fox, Phillip Corlett, Rachel Beeder, Rachel Jespersen, Randy Buckner, Richard Friedman, Ritwik Niyogi, Rob Rutledge, Ryan Smith, Sahil Garg, Sahrath Guntuku, Sarah Yip, Shaynna Herrera, Simon Eickhoff, Stanley Lyndon, Stephen Jaeger, Steve Heisig, Tom Insel, Uri Hasson, Wolfgang Tschacher, Xavier Castellanos, and Yulia Landa. (I'm sorry if we spoke and I forgot to put your name down!)

And finally, a special thank-you to my wife, Kristin Budde, MD MPH, who not only read every word in this book with a discerning eye, but juggled working as an emergency room psychiatrist during a pandemic while managing our toddler for large chunks of time so I could draft this book in just over seven months.

None of the ideas we've discussed are new. Claude Bernard was a French physician who, in the mid-1800s, first articulated the fundamental tenet of experimental medicine: measure everything. Bernard and his compatriots wanted to demonstrate to themselves that the treatments they gave their patients *actually were* helpful. To do this, they decided to measure whatever data they believed to be clinically relevant as rigorously as possible: They measured patients they treated, they measured patients they didn't treat, and then measured whether and how those two groups differed over time. Only by measuring, Bernard reasoned, could he ensure his treatments were useful; anything less might be just wishful thinking. Among other things, Bernard and colleagues invented the double-blind randomized clinical trial, which is the standard of proof still used in the medical community. Bernard's book, *An Introduction to the Study of Experimental Medicine*, describes the theoretical foundation upon which modern medical science is built.

If you want to dig a little deeper, beyond medical science, consider reading Alfred Crosby's *The Measure of Reality*, an accessible account of the shift from qualitative to quantitative thinking in Western society and why that was a milestone in advancing Western culture.

Another way of viewing the rise of quantification is as a desire to fully capture and represent reality, as described in Lorraine Daston and Peter Galison's essay (and later book), *The Image of Objectivity*. Daston and Galison argue that our concept of objectivity has changed over time, typically in connection with the development of some new technology (photograph) that supplements our senses (eye). Of interest to our discussion is how clinical studies that previously focused on snapshots of clinical outcome (or cross-sectional analyses) are now being seen as less representative of clinical reality than studies wherein data is gathered over a protracted period (longitudinal analyses).

Overall, as I alluded to in the Introduction, the reason why measurements are so crucial to medical science is because, in the absence of measurements, it's impossible to operationalize and, therefore, to mathematically evaluate and improve clinical decision. Leaving decisions to even highly skilled, experienced clinicians cannot overcome a fundamental limitation every clinician has: our own brains. Each clinician's decision-making capacity is a complex interaction of our experience, mood, implicit bias, nutritional status (did they have lunch?), time of day, general stress (how are things at home?), and interest. In his book *Thinking, Fast and Slow*, Daniel Kahneman describes how even the most highly trained brain struggles to make sound decisions.

140   An unresolved question is how to most ably pair a patient's self-report of symptoms, which represents their *personal experience* of illness, with quantitative data, which represents observable characteristics of that illness. A patient's personal experience of illness is perhaps nowhere more relevant than in psychiatry, where diseases of the brain can distort and warp the way someone perceives the world.

NOTES

INTRODUCTION

14 **"before or after lunch":**
Gladwell, Malcolm (2019). *Talking to Strangers*, Little, Brown & Co.

14 **"suffer from my implicit bias":** Kahneman, Daniel (2013). *Thinking, Fast and Slow*, Farrar, Straus and Giroux.

15 **"George Engel wrote in his 1977 seminal *Science*":** Engel, G. (1977). The need for a new medical model: a challenge for biomedicine *Science* 196(4286), 129–136. https:// dx.doi.org/10.1126/science.847460.

21 **"written extensively about the study's history":** Levy, D., Brink, S. (2006), *Change of Heart: Unraveling the Mysteries of Cardiovascular Disease*, Vintage Press.

22 **"cancer diagnosis . . . was based in anatomy":** Mukherjee, S. (2011), *The Emperor of All Maladies: A Biography of Cancer*, Scribner Press.

22 **"Daston and Galison":** Daston, L., Galison, P. (1992). "The Image of Objectivity," *Representations* 40(40), 81–128. https://dx.doi.org/10.2307 /2928741.

23 **"can be identified by the type of cells it contains":** I was a histology teaching assistant in
medical school, so permit me to geek out for a moment. Consider the enormous amount of knowledge required to make the histologic diagnosis of "breast cancer metastasis to the lung." To detect whether a cell found in the lungs looks out of place, you must first know what lung cells—all of the different types—look like. If you do conclude that a group of cells in the lungs is indeed out of place, to identify them as breast *cancer* cells indicates you have excluded the possibility that these cells are not from the colon, liver, or anywhere else in the body. So not only do you know what breast *cancer* cells look like (as opposed to healthy breast cells), but you further know what all other types of cells looks like. Histology doesn't typically strike people as being a Big Data field, but there's an awful lot of data required to correctly diagnose "breast cancer metastasis to the lung." This enormous amount of data, however, simplifies an otherwise highly complex problem: knowing which cells belong where.

23 **"Another example is the HER-2 mutation":** Bazel, R. (1998), *Her-2: The Making of Herceptin, a Revolutionary Treatment for Breast Cancer*, Random House Press.

25 **"I am forced to rely on my clinical impressions, on my intuition":** More than any other specific reason, the continued and exclusive reliance on clinical

142 impressions and intuition is why psychiatry does not function like a medical science. A fundamental part of any medical science is the supplementation of judgment with rigorous measurement of what is agreed to be clinically useful data. This has been a standard of care since the mid-1800s when French physicians like Claude Bernard promoted "experimental medicine" as a way to demonstrate that our treatments were effective; Bernard and colleagues designed what has become known as the double-blind randomized clinical trial, the standard test for any drug or therapy. "In the experimental sciences, measurement of phenomena is fundamental, since their law can be established by quantitatively determining and effect in relation to a given cause. In biology, if we wish to learn the laws of life, we must therefore not only observe and note vital phenomena [which is what I do in clinic already], but moreover also define numerically the ratios of their relative intensity one to another." (Bernard, C. [1957]. *An Introduction to the Study of Experimental Medicine*. Dover Publications, p. 129).

CHAPTER ONE

31 **"a statistic that is only expected to increase":** Torous, J., Kiang, M. V., Lorme, J., Onnela, J.-P. "New Tools for New Research in Psychiatry: A Scalable and Customizable Platform to Empower Data Driven Smartphone Research." *JMIR Mental Health* 3, e16 (2016). See also Hsin, H., Torous, J., Roberts, L. "An Adjuvant Role for Mobile Health in Psychiatry." *JAMA Psychiatry* 73, 103–104 (2016).

31 **"Every second, forty thousand people Google something":** "Google Search Statistics." https://www.internetlivestats.com/google-search-statistics/.

31 **"1.2 billion people log onto Facebook":** Shaban, Hamza, "Twitter reveals its daily active user numbers for the first time," *Washington Post*, February 7, 2019. Accessed at https://www.washingtonpost.com/technology/2019/02/07/twitter-reveals-its-daily-active-user-numbers-first-time/.

33 **"tremendously revealing":** Stephens-Davidowitz, S. *Everybody Lies*. Dey Street Books.

33 **"During the COVID-19 pandemic":** "Google Searches Can Help Us Find Emerging Covid-19 Outbreaks," Stephens-Davidowitz, S. *New York Times*, April 5, 2020. https://www.nytimes.com/2020/04/05/opinion/coronavirus-google-searches.html. Lampos, V., Moura, S., Yom-Tov, E., Edelstein, M., Majumder, M., Hamada, Y., Rangaka, M., McKendry, R., Cox, I. (2020). "Tracking COVID-19 Using Online Search," *Arxiv*. https://arxiv.org/pdf/2003.08086.pdf.

34 **"find a job"**: Baker, S., Fradkin, A. "What Drives Job Search? Evidence from Google Search Data," March 30, 2011, http://www-siepr .stanford.edu/RePEc/sip/10-020 .pdf.

34 **"vote in a presidential election"**: Stephens-Davidowitz, S. "The Cost of Racial Animus on a Black Presidential Candidate: Using Google Search Data to Find What Surveys Miss," March 24, 2013. Accessed at http://static1 .squarespace.com/static/51d894bee 4b01caf88ccb4f3/t/51d89ab3e4b05 a25fc1f39d4/1373149875469/Racial AnimusAndVotingSethStephens Davidowitz.pdf.

34 **"top ten questions"**: Stephens-Davidowitz, S. "What Do Pregnant Women Want?" *New York Times,* May 17, 2014. https:// www.nytimes.com/2014/05/18 /opinion/sunday/what-do -pregnant-women-want.html

35 **"Columbia Suicide Severity Rating Scale"**: "Columbia Suicide Severity Rating Scale" (C-SSRS), National Suicide Prevention Hotline, SAMHSA, https://suicide preventionlifeline.org/wp-content /uploads/2016/09/Suicide-Risk -Assessment-C-SSRS-Lifeline -Version-2014.pdf.

35 **"Google searches for explicitly suicidal terms were better able to predict completed suicides"**: Ma-Kellams, C., Or, F., Baek, J., Kawachi, I. (2016).

"Rethinking Suicide Surveillance." *Clinical Psychological Science* 4, 480–484.

36 **"Olga Khazan recently observed in the *Atlantic*"**: Khazan, O. "What Your Facebook Posts Say About Your Mental Health," *Atlantic,* November 6, 2019.

36 **"in the *British Medical Journal*"**: Guntuku, S., Schneider, R., Pelullo, A., Young, J., Wong, V., Ungar, L., Polsky, D., Volpp, K., Merchant, R. (2019). "Studying Expressions of Loneliness in Individuals Using Twitter: An Observational Study." *BMJ Open* 9(11), e030355 - 8. https://dx.doi .org/10.1136/bmjopen-2019 -030355. See also, Coppersmith, G., Dredze, M., Harman, C. (2014). "Quantifying Mental Health Signals in Twitter." *Proceedings of the Workshop on Computational Linguistics and Clinical Psychology: From Linguistic Signal to Clinical Reality,* 51–60 doi:10.3115/v1 /w14-3207.

39 **"they announced giving birth"**: Choudhury, M., Counts, S., Horvitz, E. (2013). "Predicting Postpartum Changes in Emotion and Behavior via Social Media." *The SIGCHI Conference,* 3267–3276 doi:10.1145/2470654.2466447.

40 **"using Facebook posts in 165 women"**: Choudhury, M., Counts, S., Horvitz, E. J., Hoff, A., Hoff, A. (2014). "Characterizing and

144 Predicting Postpartum Depression from Shared Facebook Data." *CSCW* doi:10.1145/2531602.2531675.

40 **"in the journal *Schizophrenia*":** Birnbaum, M. et al (2019). "Detecting Relapse in Youth with Psychotic Disorders Utilizing Patient-Generated and Patient-Contributed Digital Data from Facebook. *NPJ Schizophrenia* 1–9 doi:10.1038/s41537-019-0085-9.

CHAPTER TWO

47 **"difference between homosexuality and heterosexuality in any metric":** Friedman, R., Downey, J. (1994). "Homosexuality." *New England Journal of Medicine* 331(14), 923–930.

50 **"Each measure captures a facet of someone's lived experience":** Torous, J., Kiang, M., Lorme, J., Onnela, J. (2016). "New Tools for New Research in Psychiatry: A Scalable and Customizable Platform to Empower Data Driven Smartphone Research." *JMIR Mental Health* 3(2), e16. https://dx.doi.org/10.2196/mental.5165.

50 **"Accelerometers have a long history in psychiatry":** Teicher, M. (1995). "Actigraphy and Motion Analysis: New Tools for Psychiatry." *Harvard Review of Psychiatry* 3(1), 18–35. https://dx.doi.org/10.3109/10673229509017161.

50 **"explicitly to measure movement in psychiatric patients":** Teicher, M. (1995). "Actigraphy and Motion Analysis: New Tools for Psychiatry." *Harvard Review of Psychiatry* 3(1), 18–35. https://dx.doi.org/10.3109/10673229509017161.

52 **"Dr. Linda Porrino and colleagues":** Porrino, L., Rapoport, J., Behar, D., Sceery, W., Ismond, D., Bunney, W. (1983). "A Naturalistic Assessment of the Motor Activity of Hyperactive Boys," *Archives of General Psychiatry* 40(6), 681. https://dx.doi.org/10.1001/archpsyc.1983.04390010091012.

52 **"bringing this hyperactivity to normal":** Porrino, L., Rapoport, J., Behar, D., Ismond, D., Bunney, W. (1983). "A Naturalistic Assessment of the Motor Activity of Hyperactive Boys," *Archives of General Psychiatry* 40(6), 688. https://dx.doi.org/10.1001/archpsyc.1983.04390010098013.

54 **"Your Apps Know Where You Were Last Night":** Valentino-DeVries, J., Singer, N., Keller, M., Krolick, A. "Your Apps Know Where You Were Last Night, and They're Not Keeping It Secret," *New York Times*, December 10, 2018. https://www.nytimes.com/interactive/2018/12/10/business/location-data-privacy-apps.html.

55 **"people who used the app were less likely to drink alcohol":** Gustafson, D., McTavish, F.,

Chih, M., Atwood, A., Johnson, R., Boyle, M., Levy, M., Driscoll, H., Chisholm, S., Dillenburg, L., Isham, A., Shah, D. (2014). "A Smartphone Application to Support Recovery From Alcoholism: A Randomized Clinical Trial." *JAMA Psychiatry* 71(5), 566–572. https://dx.doi.org /10.1001/jamapsychiatry.2013.4642.

56 **"to model how information or disease would spread through this social network":** Kim, D., Hwong, A., Stafford, D., Hughes, D., O'Malley, A., Fowler, J., Christakis, N. (2015). "Social Network Targeting to Maximise Population Behaviour Change: A Cluster Randomised Controlled Trial." *Lancet* 386(9989), 145–153. https:// dx.doi.org/10.1016/s0140-6736 (15)60095-2.

56–57 **"built a social network from millions of mobile call logs over an eighteen-week period":** Onnela, J., Saramaki, J., Hyvonen, J., Szabo, G., Lazer, D., Kaski, K., Kertesz, J., Barabasi, A. (2006). "Structure and Tie Strengths in Mobile Communication Networks." *Proceedings of the National Academy of Sciences* 104(18), 7332–7336. https://dx.doi.org/10.1073/pnas .0610245104

CHAPTER THREE

63 **"habit has made us blind to our own vague inadequacy":** I have observed that some clinicians do indeed believe that, simply by speaking with a patient for fifteen or twenty minutes, they feel they have all the data they need to make treatment decisions. I have stood quietly during discussions about patients where clinicians discuss which neurotransmitters are "depleted" or perhaps need to be "augmented"—as if speaking with their patient was a window into their neurotransmitter function. Perhaps worse, some clinicians really get into the weeds about specific neurotransmitter receptors, discussing how one medication (e.g., escitalopram) is a less optimal treatment than another (e.g., bupropion) for a particular patient based on the *receptor profile*; as if they know what a given patient's receptor profile is after a simple conversation. This is simply ridiculous.

65 **" a response to the total stimulus situation before the reagent":** Sanford, F. (1942). "Speech and Personality." *Psychological Bulletin* 39(10), 811–845.

66 **"Silhouettes swaying at the hips might be feminine whereas blockish silhouettes might be masculine":** To get more of an intuition for how movement can express emotion and for how movement can be measured, I encourage you to play with the interactive program found at http:// www.biomotionlab.ca/Demos /BMLwalker.html.

146

69   "a computer program they wrote performed a task that would take one person working full-time eight months": Jong, N., Wempe, T. (2009). "Praat Script to Detect Syllable Nuclei and Measure Speech Rate Automatically." *Behavior Research Methods* 41(2), 385–390. https://dx.doi.org/10.3758/brm .41.2.385.

73   "these patterns can be used to predict eventual psychosis": Bedi, G., Carrillo, F., Cecchi, G., Slezak, D., Sigman, M., Mota, N., Ribeiro, S., Javitt, D., Copelli, M., Corcoran, C. (2015). "Automated Analysis of Free Speech Predicts Psychosis Onset in High-Risk Youths." *NPJ Schizophrenia* 1(1), 15030. https:// dx.doi.org/10.1038 /npjschz.2015.30.

74   "speech could be used to predict a psychotic episode with up to 82 percent accuracy": Corcoran, C., Carrillo, F., Fernández-Slezak, D., Bedi, G., Klim, C., Javitt, D., Bearden, C., Cecchi, G. (2018). "Prediction of Psychosis Across Protocols and Risk Cohorts Using Automated Language Analysis." *World Psychiatry* 17(1), 67–75. https:// dx.doi.org/10.1002/wps.20491.

75   "reflected the quality and outcome of their therapeutic relationship": Ramseyer, F., Tschacher, W. (2011). "Nonverbal Synchrony in Psychotherapy: Coordinated Body Movement Reflects Relationship Quality and Outcome." *Journal of Consulting and Clinical Psychology* 79(3), 284–295. https://dx.doi.org/10.1037 /a0023419.

75   "an *embodiment* of emotion": Tschacher, W., Giersch, A., Friston, K. (2017). "Embodiment and Schizophrenia: A Review of Implications and Applications." *Schizophrenia Bulletin* 43(4), 745– 753. https://dx.doi.org/10.1093 /schbul/sbw220.

CHAPTER FOUR

80   "by sampling the world": Friston, K. (2010). "The Free-Energy Principle: A Unified Brain Theory?" *Nature Reviews Neuroscience* 11(2), 127–138. https://dx.doi.org/10.1038 /nrn2787.

81   "to compare these guesses to what we see, hear, and feel": Friston, K. (2018). "Does Predictive Coding Have a Future?" *Nature Neuroscience* 21(8), 1019–1021. https://dx.doi.org/10.1038 /s41593-018-0200-7.

84   "often tearing it apart": Barron, D. (2018). "Can We Measure Delusions?" *Scientific American*. Much of this section is based on this piece.

85   "models that—if we view the brain as an inference machine— underlie hallucinations":

Powers, A., Mathys, C., Corlett, P. (2017). "Pavlovian Conditioning-Induced Hallucinations Result from Overweighting of Perceptual Priors." *Science* 357(6351), 596–600. https://dx.doi.org/10.1126/science.aan3458.

87 "Experimental evidence in a group of nearly twenty thousand people shows this is indeed the case": Rutledge, R., Skandali, N., Dayan, P., Dolan, R. (2014). "A Computational and Neural Model of Momentary Subjective Well-Being." *Proceedings of the National Academy of Sciences* 111(33), 12252-12257. https://dx.doi.org/10.1073/pnas.1407535111.

88 "set you on a path toward an elevated mood": Mason, L., Eldar, E., Rutledge, R. (2017). "Mood Instability and Reward Dysregulation—A Neurocomputational Model of Bipolar Disorder." *JAMA Psychiatry* 74(12), 1275–2. https://dx.doi.org/10.1001/jamapsychiatry.2017.3163.

88 "crescendo into a positive mood as an escalatory cycle": Eldar, E., Rutledge, R., Dolan, R., Niv, Y. (2016). "Mood as Representation of Momentum." *Trends in Cognitive Sciences* 20(1), 15–24. https://dx.doi.org/10.1016/j.tics.2015.07.010.

88 "might lead to bipolar disorder": Mason, L., Eldar,

E., Rutledge, R. (2017). "Mood Instability and Reward Dysregulation—A Neurocomputational Model of Bipolar Disorder." *JAMA Psychiatry* 74(12), 1275–2. https://dx.doi.org/10.1001/jamapsychiatry.2017.3163.

89 "Anxiety is extremely common": Barron, D. (2018). "Is Chronic Anxiety a Learning Disorder?" *Scientific American.*

89 "participants tried to win a pot of money": Behrens, T., Woolrich, M., Walton, M., Rushworth, M. (2007). "Learning the Value of Information in an Uncertain World." *Nature Neuroscience* 10(9), 1214–1221. https://dx.doi.org/10.1038/nn1954.

90 "get an electric zap if you choose incorrectly": Browning, M., Behrens, T., Jocham, G., O'Reilly, J., Bishop, S. (2015). "Anxious Individuals Have Difficulty Learning the Causal Statistics of Aversive Environments." *Nature Neuroscience* 18(4), 590–596. https://dx.doi.org/10.1038/nn.3961.

CHAPTER FIVE

94 "to make sense of human suffering": Harrington, A. (2019). *Mind Fixers: Psychiatry's Troubled Search for the Biology of Mental Illness.* W.W. Norton & Company.

95 "270 million unique combinations of symptoms":

148 Allsopp, K., Read, J., Corcoran, R., Kinderman, P. (2019). "Heterogeneity in Psychiatric Diagnostic Classification." *Psychiatry Research* 279, 15–22. https://dx.doi.org/10.1016/j.psychres.2019.07.005.

96 **"why it was designed"**: Clarke, D., Narrow, W., Regier, D., Kuramoto, S., Kupfer, D., Kuhl, E., Greiner, L., Kraemer, H. (2013). "DSM-5 Field Trials in the United States and Canada, Part I: Study Design, Sampling Strategy, Implementation, and Analytic Approaches." *American Journal of Psychiatry* 170(1), 43–58. https://dx.doi.org/10.1176/appi.ajp.2012.12070998. See also: Regier, D., Narrow, W., Clarke, D., Kraemer, H., Kuramoto, S., Kuhl, E., Kupfer, D. (2013). "DSM-5 Field Trials in the United States and Canada, Part II: Test-Retest Reliability of Selected Categorical Diagnoses." *American Journal of Psychiatry* 170(1), 59–70. https://dx.doi.org/10.1176/appi.ajp.2012.12070999.

98 **"try to predict a given clinical variable"**: Barron, D., Bzdok, D., Krystal, J., Constable, R. (2020). "What Can Machine Learning Do for Psychiatry?" *Biological Psychiatry* 87(9), S462. https://dx.doi.org/10.1016/j.biopsych.2020.02.1176.

101 **"useful in making sense of the data produced in phenotyping"**: Friston, K., Redish, A., Gordon, J. (2017).

"Computational Nosology and Precision Psychiatry." *Computational Psychiatry* 1, 2–23. https://dx.doi.org/10.1162/cpsy_a_00001. See also: Schwartenbeck, P., Friston, K. (2016). "Computational Phenotyping in Psychiatry: A Worked Example." *eNeuro* 3(4), ENEURO.0049-16.2016. https://dx.doi.org/10.1523/eneuro.0049-16.2016.

104 **"there is not a single psychiatric disorder"**: Barron, D., Krystal, J., in preparation.

CHAPTER SIX

113 **"Beiwe platform seeks to bridge"**: Torous, J., Kiang, M., Lorme, J., Onnela, J. (2016). "New Tools for New Research in Psychiatry: A Scalable and Customizable Platform to Empower Data Driven Smartphone Research." *JMIR Mental Health* 3(2), e16. https://dx.doi.org/10.2196/mental.5165.

117 **"iOS users make $85,000"**: https://www.comscore.com/ita/Public-Relations/Infographics/iPhone-Users-Earn-Higher-Income-Engage-More-on-Apps-than-Android-Users.

117 **"Who owns what is a contentious issue in science"**: Barron, D. (2018). "How Freely Should Scientists Share Their Data?" *Scientific American*.

117 **"an opinion about data and software ownership"**: For a highly accessible overview of digital data ownership, see Doctorow, C. "Information Doesn't Want to Be Free: Laws for the Internet Age," McSweeney's Publishing, 2015.

122 **"leaving his NIMH directorship"**: Dobbs, D. "The Smartphone Psychiatrist," *Atlantic*, July/August 2017. Accessed at https://www.theatlantic.com /magazine/archive/2017/07/the -smartphone-psychiatrist/528726/.

123 **"OneFifteen is a tech-enabled, nonprofit recovery ecosystem"**: See OneFifteen History at http://onefifteen.org /about/.

126 **"discharged from the hospital"**: Fischer, E., Dornelas, E., Goethe, J. (2001). "Characteristics of People Lost to Attrition in Psychiatric Follow-up Studies." *The Journal of Nervous and Mental Disease* 189(1).

127 **"uninstall it within the first two weeks"**: Renn, B., Pratap, A., Atkins, D., Mooney, S., Areán, P. (2018). "Smartphone-Based Passive Assessment of Mobility in Depression: Challenges and Opportunities." *Mental Health and Physical Activity* 14, 136–139. https://dx.doi.org/10.1016/j .mhpa.2018.04.003.

127 **"a recent study published in *JAMA Network Open*"**: Carlo, A., Ghomi, R., Renn, B., Strong, M., Areán, P. (2020). "Assessment of Real-World Use of Behavioral Health Mobile Applications by a Novel Stickiness Metric." *JAMA Network Open* 3(8), e2011978. https://dx.doi.org/10.1001 /jamanetworkopen.2020.11978.

CONCLUSION

132 **"Google first used search records to trace flu outbreaks"**: Ginsberg, J., Mohebbi, M., Patel, R., Brammer, L., Smolinski, M., Brilliant, L. (2009). "Detecting Influenza Epidemics Using Search Engine Query Data," *Nature* 457, doi:10.1038/nature07634 http:// dx.doi.org/10.1038/nature07634. Also available at: http://static .googleusercontent.com/media /research.google.com/en/us/archive /papers/detecting-influenza -epidemics.pdf.

132 **"People embraced geolocation data"**: Fowler, G. "Smartphone Data Reveal Which Americans Are Social Distancing (And Not)," *Washington Post*, March 24, 2020. Accessed at https://www.washingtonpost.com /technology/2020/03/24/social -distancing-maps-cellphone -location/; See also, Schechner, S., Winkler, R. "Here's How Apple and Google Plan to Track the Coronavirus Through Your Phone," *Wall Street Journal,* April 11, 2020. Accessed at https://www.wsj .com/articles/heres-how-apple

150   -and-google-plan-to-track-the
-coronavirus-through-your-phone
-11586618075?mod=searchresults
&page=1&pos=14.

132   **"I can't smell"**: Stephens-
Davidowitz, S. "Google Searches
Can Help Us Find Emerging Covid-
19 Outbreaks," *New York Times*,
April 5, 2020. Accessed at https://
www.nytimes.com/2020
/04/05/opinion/coronavirus-google
-searches.html.

135   **"5.5 percent of overall
healthcare expenses"**: See https://
store.samhsa.gov/sites/default/files
/d7/priv/sma14-4883.pdf.

Columbia Global Reports is a publishing imprint from Columbia University that commissions authors to do original on-site reporting around the globe on a wide range of issues. The resulting novella-length books offer new ways to look at and understand the world that can be read in a few hours. Most readers are curious and busy. Our books are for them.